Arthroscopy and Endoscopy

Editor

REBECCA A. CERRATO

FOOT AND
ANKLE CLINICS

www.foot.theclinics.com

Consulting Editor
MARK S. MYERSON

March 2015 • Volume 20 • Number 1

ELSEVIER

1600 John F. Kennedy Boulevard • Suite 1800 • Philadelphia, Pennsylvania, 19103-2899

http://www.theclinics.com

FOOT AND ANKLE CLINICS Volume 20, Number 1
March 2015 ISSN 1083-7515, ISBN-13: 978-0-323-35655-8

Editor: Jennifer Flynn-Briggs
Developmental Editor: Meredith Clinton

Foot and Ankle Clinics (ISSN 1083-7515) is published quarterly by Elsevier, Inc., 360 Park Avenue South, New York, NY 10010-1710. Months of issue are March, June, September, and December. Periodicals postage paid at New York, NY, and additional mailing offices. Subscription price per year is $315.00 (US individuals), $421.00 (US institutions), $155.00 (US students), $360.00 (Canadian individuals), $506.00 (Canadian institutions), $215.00 (Canadian students), $460.00 (international individuals), $506.00 (international institutions), and $215.00 (international students). To receive student/resident rate, orders must be accompanied by name of affiliated institution, date of term, and the *signature* of program/residency coordinator on institution letterhead. Orders will be billed at individual rate until proof of status is received. Foreign air speed delivery is included in all *Clinics* subscription prices. All prices are subject to change without notice. **POSTMASTER:** Send address changes to *Foot and Ankle Clinics*, Elsevier Health Sciences Division, Subscription Customer Service, 3251 Riverport Lane, Maryland Heights, MO 63043. **Customer Service: 1-800-654-2452 (US and Canada). From outside of the United States and Canada, call 314-447-8871. Fax: 314-447-8029. E-mail: JournalsCustomerService-usa@ elsevier.com (for print support); JournalsOnlineSupport-usa@elsevier.com (for online support).**

Reprints. For copies of 100 or more, of articles in this publication, please contact the Commercial Reprints Department, Elsevier Inc., 360 Park Avenue South, New York, NY 10010-1710. Tel.: 212-633-3874; Fax: 212-633-3820; E-mail: reprints@elsevier.com.

Contributors

CONSULTING EDITOR

MARK S. MYERSON, MD
Director, The Institute for Foot and Ankle Reconstruction, Mercy Medical Center, Mercy Hospital, Baltimore, Maryland

EDITOR

REBECCA A. CERRATO, MD
Institute for Foot and Ankle Reconstruction, Mercy Medical Center, Mercy Hospital, Baltimore, Maryland

AUTHORS

JORGE I. ACEVEDO, MD
Southeast Orthopedic Specialists, Jacksonville, Florida

ANNUNZIATO AMENDOLA, MD
Department of Orthopaedics and Rehabilitation, University of Iowa Hospitals and Clinics, University of Iowa, Iowa City, Iowa

ALICIA BALLARD, DO
Orthopedic Department, Broward Health, Fort Lauderdale, Florida

BRANDEE S. BLACK, MD, MEd
Department of Orthopaedic Surgery, University of Missouri, Columbia, Missouri

DAVIDE EDOARDO BONASIA, MD
Department of Orthopaedics and Traumatology, AO Città della Salute e della Scienza – Presidio CTO, University of Torino, Torino, Italy

DOMINIC CARREIRA, MD
Attending Physician of Orthopedic Surgery, Orthopedics and Sports Medicine, Broward Health, Clinical Instructor of NOVA Southeastern University, Fort Lauderdale, Florida

SERGIO ECKHOLT, MD
Departamento de Ortopedia y Traumatologia, Clinica Las Condes, Santiago, Chile

ANNA O. ELMLUND, PhD
Senior Clinical Fellow, Avon Orthopaedic Centre, Southmead Hospital, Westbury-on-Trym, Bristol, United Kingdom

DAVID M. EPSTEIN, MD
Attending Staff, Morristown Medical Center, Morristown; Tri-County Orthopedics & Sports Medicine, Cedar Knolls, New Jersey

JOERG JEROSCH, MD, PhD
Prof.Dr.med.Dr.h.c., Department of Orthopedic Surgery and Sports Medicine,
Johanna-Etienne-Hospital, Neuss, Germany

TUN HING LUI, MBBS (HK), FRCS (Edin), FHKAM, FHKCOS
Consultant, Department of Orthopaedics and Traumatology, North District Hospital, Hong
Kong, China

ERNESTO MACEIRA, MD
Orthopaedic Foot and Ankle Unit, Orthopaedic and Trauma Department, Hospital
Universitario Quirón Madrid, Madrid, Spain

PETER MANGONE, MD
Director, Foot and Ankle Services; Co-Director, Foot and Ankle Center, Blue Ridge Bone
and Joint Clinic, Mission Hospital, Asheville, North Carolina

TAKASHI MATSUSHITA, MD
Department of Orthopaedic Surgery, Teikyo University School of Medicine, Tokyo, Japan

WATARU MIYAMOTO, MD
Department of Orthopaedic Surgery, Teikyo University School of Medicine, Tokyo, Japan

MANUEL MONTEAGUDO, MD
Faculty of Medicine, Universidad Europea de Madrid; Orthopaedic Foot and Ankle Unit,
Orthopaedic and Trauma Department, Hospital Universitario Quirón Madrid, Madrid,
Spain

GERARDO MUÑOZ, MD, PhD
Departamento de Ortopedia y Traumatologia, Clinica Las Condes, Santiago, Chile

PHINIT PHISITKUL, MD
Department of Orthopaedics and Rehabilitation, University of Iowa Hospitals and Clinics,
University of Iowa, Iowa City, Iowa

MARCO PIRAS, MD
Orthopedic Department, Nuovo Ospedale degli Infermi, Biella, ASLBI, Piemonte, Italy

SETH L. SHERMAN, MD
Assistant Professor of Orthopedic Surgery, Department of Orthopaedic Surgery,
University of Missouri, Columbia, Missouri

ALBERTO SICLARI, MD
Orthopedic Department, Nuovo Ospedale degli Infermi, Biella, ASLBI, Piemonte, Italy

MASATO TAKAO, MD
Department of Orthopaedic Surgery, Teikyo University School of Medicine, Tokyo, Japan

LUNG FUNG TSE, FHKAM, FHKCOS
Associate Consultant, Department of Orthopaedics and Traumatology, Prince of Wales
Hospital, Hong Kong, China

IAN G. WINSON, FRCS
Consultant Orthopaedic Surgeon, Avon Orthopaedic Centre, Southmead Hospital,
Westbury-on-Trym, Bristol, United Kingdom

CHI PAN YUEN, MBBS (HK), FRCS (Edin), FHKAM
Specialist Resident, Department of Orthopaedics and Traumatology, Kwong Wah
Hospital, Hong Kong, China

Contents

 Videos of posterior tibial tendon tendoscopy accompany this article

> The posterior tibial tendon (PTT) helps the triceps surae to work more efficiently during ambulation. Disorders of the PTT include tenosynovitis, acute rupture, degenerative tears, dislocation, instability, enthesopathies, and chronic tendinopathy with dysfunction and flat foot deformity. Open surgery of the PTT has been the conventional approach to deal with these disorders. However, tendoscopy has become a useful technique to diagnose and treat PTT disorders. This article focuses on PTT tendoscopy and tries to provide an understanding of the pathomechanics of the tendon, indications for surgery, surgical technique, advantages, complications, and limitations of this procedure.

> Peroneal tendoscopy is indicated for peroneal tenosynovitis, subluxation or dislocation, snapping, partial tears requiring debridement, and postoperative adhesions and scarring. Peroneal tendoscopy was also found to be valuable as a diagnostic tool in some instances. It is generally reported to have good to excellent outcomes in most patients with a relatively low occurrence of complications.

 Videos of endoscopic gastrocnemius release and endoscopic treatment for Haglund's deformity accompany this article

> Endoscopic surgery provides a minimally invasive approach to visualize and treat several pathologic conditions of the Achilles tendon. Open surgery on the Achilles tendon is notorious for wound complications, whereas endoscopic procedures have been recognized for less scaring, less perioperative pain, fewer wound complications, and faster recovery. This article reviews various endoscopic techniques for the treatment of equinus contracture, Achilles rupture, Haglund's deformity, and noninsertional Achilles tendinopathy.

> Anterior ankle arthroscopy is a useful, minimally invasive technique for diagnosing and treating ankle conditions. Arthroscopic treatment offers

the benefit of decreased surgical morbidity, less postoperative pain, and earlier return to activities. Indications for anterior ankle arthroscopy continue to expand, including ankle instability, impingement, management of osteochondritis dissecans, synovectomy, and loose body removal. Anterior ankle arthroscopy has its own set of inherent risks and complications. Surgeons can decrease the risk of complications through mastery of ankle anatomy and biomechanics, and by careful preoperative planning and meticulous surgical technique.

The emergence of subtalar arthroscopy has improved the understanding and accuracy of diagnosing several hindfoot pathologic conditions, in particular, sinus tarsi syndrome. Subtalar arthroscopy has evolved into a useful diagnostic and therapeutic tool. The surgeon's experience is still essential to achieve good results. This article reviews the clinical indications, surgical techniques, and outcomes of subtalar arthroscopy.

With mounting attention focused on decreasing postsurgical pain and dysfunction, emphasis has been placed on approaching disorders using minimally invasive techniques. Surgical procedures of the hallux, such as hallux valgus correction, have earned the reputation for high postsurgical pain and prolonged recovery. Arthroscopic hallux procedures have the advantages of minimizing pain, swelling, and disability. Certain conditions, such as synovitis, loose bodies, and early-grade hallux rigidus, are better addressed arthroscopically. With the correct indications, hallux metatarsophalangeal arthroscopy can be a valuable tool for the foot and ankle surgeon.

The clinical application of small joint arthroscopies (metatarsophalangeal joint, Lisfranc joint, Chopart joint, and interphlangeal joint) in the foot has seen significant advancements in the past decades. This article reviews the clinical indications, technical details, outcomes, and potential complications of small joint arthroscopies of the foot.

 Videos of resections of the flexor hallucis longus tendon accompany this article

Hindfoot endoscopic surgery is an alternative to conventional open surgery for treatment of posterior ankle pain. This procedure can be applied not only for accurate diagnosis under direct visualization but also for low-invasive therapy. Common indications for hindfoot endoscopy are posterior ankle impingement syndrome and damaged soft tissue. Several studies have reported good clinical outcomes of hindfoot endoscopy with lower complication rates than in the conventional open procedure. Nerve injury remains a common complication. To avoid such injury, make a posterolateral portal just lateral to the Achilles tendon and perform the hindfoot endoscopic procedure in the region lateral to the flexor hallucis longus tendon.

Joerg Jerosch

> Opinions differ regarding the surgical treatment of posterior calcaneal exostosis. After failure of conservative treatment, open surgical bursectomy and resection of the calcaneal prominence is indicated by many investigators. Clinical studies have shown high rates of unsatisfactory results and complications. Endoscopic calcaneoplasty (ECP) is a minimally invasive surgical option that can avoid some of these obstacles. ECP is an effective procedure for the treatment of patients with posterior calcaneal exostosis. The endoscopic exposure is superior to the open technique and has less morbidity, less operating time, fewer complications, and the disorders can be better differentiated.

FOOT AND ANKLE CLINICS

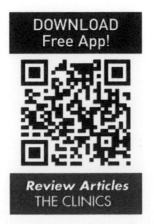

Preface
Current Techniques and Future Direction

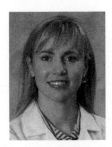

Rebecca A. Cerrato, MD
Editor

Arthroscopy of the foot and ankle has evolved from simply a diagnostic tool to a versatile treatment modality for a variety of pathologic abnormalities. With the reputation of prolonged swelling and higher wound complication risks, the benefits of performing these foot and ankle procedures through a minimally invasive approach is evident. In addition, advancements in small joint arthroscopes and instrumentation have provided surgeons the tools to effectively expand their indications. This issue of *Foot and Ankle Clinics of North America* presents various arthroscopic techniques and their results, reviewing established surgical procedures, while discussing several newer ones.

A diverse, international group of experts has contributed to this issue. These authors discuss current techniques, indications, and outcomes involving ankle, hindfoot, and forefoot arthroscopy, tendoscopy of the peroneals, Achilles and posterior tibial tendons, and endoscopic procedures for various conditions such as Haglund syndrome.

I would like to thank all the authors for their contributions to this issue. I would also like to thank my mentor and partner, Dr Mark Myerson, Consulting Editor for *Foot and Ankle Clinics of North America*, for inviting me to serve as guest editor for this issue. The authors and I hope this issue introduces several new arthroscopic techniques, while stimulating further debate and interest in minimally invasive foot and ankle surgery.

Rebecca A. Cerrato, MD
Institute for Foot and Ankle Reconstruction
Mercy Medical Center
Mercy Hospital
301 St. Paul Place
Baltimore, MD 21202, USA

E-mail address:
rcerrato@mdmercy.com

Foot Ankle Clin N Am 20 (2015) xi
http://dx.doi.org/10.1016/j.fcl.2014.12.001
1083-7515/15/$ – see front matter © 2015 Published by Elsevier Inc.

foot.theclinics.com

Posterior Tibial Tendoscopy

Manuel Monteagudo, MD[a,b,*], Ernesto Maceira, MD[a]

KEYWORDS

- Tendoscopy • Posterior tibial tendon • Endoscopy • Adult flatfoot

KEY POINTS

- Disorders of posterior tibial tendon (PTT) include tenosynovitis, acute rupture, degenerative tears, dislocation, instability, enthesopathies, and chronic tendinopathy with dysfunction and flat foot deformity.
- Open surgery was the conventional approach to deal with these disorders.
- Tendoscopy offers advantages over open procedures. There are fewer wound infections, and smaller wounds; in addition, there is less morbidity, quicker recovery, early mobilization and function, mild postoperative pain, and the possibility of being performed under local anesthesia on an outpatient basis.
- PTT tendoscopy allows for the visualization and palpation of the tendon, the tendon sheath, the vinculum, and partial tears.
- Tendoscopy may be the gold standard technique to perform adhesiolysis, synovectomy, debridement of partial tears, and restore physiologic gliding properties of the PTT, with low complication rates.

Videos of posterior tibial tendon tendoscopy accompany this article at http://www.foot.theclinics.com/

INTRODUCTION

Proper function of posterior tibial tendon (PTT) may be impaired by direct or indirect trauma, systemic inflammatory diseases, flatfoot deformity, or iatrogenic causes.

Imaging studies may suggest the type and location of injury, but there are several false-positive and false-negative studies. An inherent drawback of MRI is the difficulty to categorize PTT abnormalities. Inhomogeneity of the tendon on MRI could be due to tendinopathy, partial tear, degeneration, or reactive synovitis.

The authors have nothing to disclose.

[a] Orthopaedic Foot and Ankle Unit, Orthopaedic and Trauma Department, Hospital Universitario Quirón Madrid, Calle Diego de Velázquez n°1, 28223 Pozuelo de Alarcón, Madrid, Spain; [b] Universidad Europea de Madrid, C/Tajo s/n, Villaviciosa de Odón, Madrid 28670, Spain
* Corresponding author.
E-mail address: mmontyr@yahoo.com

Foot Ankle Clin N Am 20 (2015) 1–13
http://dx.doi.org/10.1016/j.fcl.2014.10.009
1083-7515/15/$ – see front matter © 2015 Elsevier Inc. All rights reserved.

Open surgery is frequently needed to establish a diagnosis and to treat PTT disorders that have not responded to conservative treatments. However, open surgery has not been free of complications such as adhesions and painful scars. Over the last decade, tendoscopy has become a useful tool to diagnose and treat tendon disorders by providing a dynamic anatomic assessment of certain tendons and pathologic entities. Most indications for open surgery of the PTT are now covered by PTT tendoscopy with less morbidity and faster return to daily activities including sport.

ANATOMY

The PTT is the largest and most anterior tendon in the posterior ankle retinaculum. The muscle is contained within the deep posterior compartment of the leg, originating on the tibia, the interosseous membrane, and the fibula, and it descends within the posterior compartment of the leg.[1] The synovial sheath of the PTT is 7 to 9 cm in length and starts around 6 cm proximal to the tip of the medial malleolus. It descends along the tendon in the retromalleolar groove, with a shift in direction of almost 90° around the medial malleolus, and it terminates close to the tuberosity of the navicular.[2] When the tendon enters the foot, it flattens, and the tissue structure changes. It exhibits an increased amount of fibrocartilage.[3,4] Histochemical studies have shown hypovascularization of the PTT in the retromalleolar region,[5,6] but another study did not confirm that extent.[7] PTT has no mesotendon, but it has a vinculum (specialized form of mesotendon), which is consistently found on the posterior side of the tendon, between the posterior side of the PTT and most posterior side of the sheath.[1] It runs in all directions proximally to end with a free edge at around 4.3 cm (range 3.5–6.5 cm) above the posteromedial tip of the medial malleolus. The vinculum is irrigated by vessels from the posterior tibial artery collaterals, running from the flexor digitorum longus synovium.[8] It is important to respect this vinculum when establishing the proximal portal for tendoscopy.

PATHOMECHANICS

The posterior tibial muscle/tendon is physiologically stretched during the first rocker of gait to allow subtalar pronation.[9] During the second rocker of gait, the PTT helps to center the talus over the navicular. Transition from the second to the third rocker starts at heel lift. The PTT actively externally rotates the tibia/leg and induces foot supination. During the third rocker, the foot behaves like a wheelbarrow, which is balanced by the peroneal tendons and the PTT. The PTT allows for the locking of the medial column of the foot during the third rocker, by the lock of the calcaneus to the cuboid and the talus to the navicular.

The PTT is a gliding tendon as it changes direction by curving around the medial malleolus. Fibrocartilage found within connective tissue is due to repetitive stimulus of intermittent compressive and shear forces.[10] The fibrocartilaginous region of PTT is located around the medial malleolus and is more vulnerable to repetitive microtrauma. It is in this region where most ruptures occur. Degeneration may arise because of the poor repair response of the hypovascular fibrocartilaginous tissue. This portion of the tendon rubs back and forth between the underlying malleolus and the overlying flexor digitorum longus. Longitudinal friction and changes in the gliding resistance of the tendon make PTT more susceptible to suffering longitudinal tears.[10]

The sliding properties of PTT may be altered due to synovitis, an irregular medial malleolus, longitudinal or transverse splits, elongation because of continuous overpronation, or a combination of several disorders. All these entities may lead to fibrous tissue formation between the tendon and the surrounding synovial sheath. Secondary neovascularization and neoinnervation may be a cause of pain in PTT tendinopathy.[11]

CLINICAL EXAMINATION

Patients suffering from PTT disorders usually present with posteromedial ankle pain. Visual gait analysis will be of help to appreciate excessive hindfoot valgus. In post-traumatic and systemic inflammatory cases there may be a normal hindfoot axis. Swelling may be present around the medial malleolus and tenderness on palpation usually located from the tip of the malleolus to the navicular (**Fig. 1**). Weakness of supination is usually encountered on manual testing of the muscle (inversion strength of the hindfoot by plantar flexed ankle). In post-traumatic cases, it is important to take notice of scars to plan portal placement.

IMAGING STUDIES

Plain radiographs with weight-bearing dorsoplantar and lateral views reveal hindfoot alignment and may allow for the evaluation of a PTT disorder in cases of flatfoot deformity or hypertrophic changes at the navicular attachment. Post-traumatic changes around the medial malleolus (fracture malunion or nonunion), subluxation of the ankle, or any possible arthritis may also be observed.

Ultrasound is useful for the assessment of the integrity of the PTT, visualization of tendon fibers, dynamic properties, and tenderness to sonopalpation. Associated hypervascularity on color Doppler and thickening of the peritendinous tissues may suggest tendinopathy. Partial or total ruptures may also be diagnosed sonographically. Dynamic assessment of PTT in the retromalleolar groove may reveal subluxation or dislocation out of a shallow or irregular groove.[12]

Rosenberg and colleagues[13] reported on the correlation of computed tomography (CT) and surgical findings in ruptures of the PTT. Although CT findings were accurate in 96% of patients who underwent surgery, 14% of ruptures were underestimated in terms of the extent of injury, so certain ruptures were misclassified.

MRI is considered the gold standard for the study of PTT disorders. MRI is helpful for assessing soft tissue abnormalities, bony changes, and bone edema. Longitudinal tears of the PTT that can be identified on MRI that are sometimes difficult to reveal in open surgery.[14] Tendoscopy may be helpful in identifying these longitudinal tears by careful palpation of the tendon with a probe.

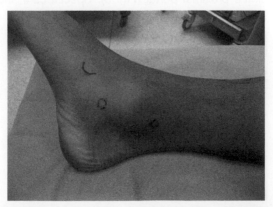

Fig. 1. Clinical examination reveals swollen PTT around the medial malleolus.

POSTERIOR TIBIAL TENDON TENDOSCOPY

PTT tendoscopy was first performed by Wertheimer in 1994,[15] although it was van Dijk who described the procedure in detail.[16] Tendoscopy is considered when all conservative treatments fail to achieve a painless and functional ankle.

Surgical Technique

With the patient supine and a tourniquet in the thigh, references are marked on the skin to identify the navicular, the PTT, the medial malleolus, and the 2 main portals (**Fig. 2**). Inversion and eversion of the foot may facilitate the identification of anatomic landmarks.

For conventional PTT tendoscopy, the equipment required is fairly basic. It is recommended to use a 2.7 mm scope with an inclination angle of 30° to facilitate access to the tendon, but a 4.0 mm arthroscope may be used for most PTT tendoscopies. A high-pressure inflow circuit may be created by having the saline bags at the highest possible level in the operating room.

Two portals are usually recommended, between 1.5 and 2 cm proximal and distal to the tip of the medial malleolus.[16] Reilingh modified the portals, by placing skin incisions between 2 and 3 cm away from the tip of the medial malleolus.[17] Recently, Roussignol has described an accessory third portal placed 7 cm proximal to the medial malleolus, in order to gain access to explore the complete PTT from the myotendinous junction.[8]

The procedure may be performed under general, regional, or local anesthesia.

The distal portal is created first. A 1 cm skin incision is made over the PTT, halfway between the medial malleolus and the navicular following the longitudinal axis of the tendon. Subcutaneous dissection is made to expose PTT sheath. The sheath is opened with a 1 cm incision perpendicular to the longitudinal axis of the tendon. This crossed disposition between the skin and the tendon sheath incisions is useful to prevent unintentionally enlarging the entry to the tendon when moving the scope during surgery (**Fig. 3**). The arthroscope with blunt trocar is introduced, and the tendon sheath is inspected without saline to gain information on synovitis. Following dry inspection, the sheath is filled with saline. While inverting the foot, the arthroscope is advanced carefully to inspect the complete PTT up to the vinculum, at around 4 cm proximal to the tip of the medial malleolus (Video 1).

The proximal portal is placed around 3 cm proximally to the tip of the medial malleolus (**Fig. 4**). Under direct visualization, the insertion of a spinal needle helps to place the skin incision for the proximal portal (**Fig. 5**). Special care should be taken to

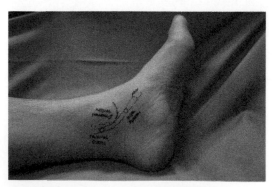

Fig. 2. References are marked on the skin prior to tendoscopy.

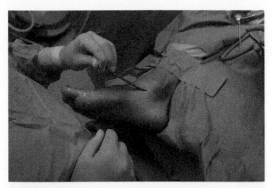

Fig. 3. Distal portal is made to gain access to the tendon.

orientate the needle and the scalpel obliquely so as not to penetrate and damage the tendon (Video 2). With the arthroscope in the distal portal, a blunt probe and a shaver system may be introduced through the proximal portal (**Fig. 6**). The complete tendon sheath can be inspected by rotating the scope around the tendon (Video 3).

A more proximal third portal, at around 7 cm from the medial malleolus, may be created in cases of severe synovitis when subtotal synovectomy proximally may also be needed.

At the end of the procedure, portals are closed with absorbable sutures. A compression bandage is recommended for the first 24 hours, and then an adhesive bandage is used to cover skin incisions. Weight bearing is allowed as tolerated immediately after surgery (provided associated procedures do not require to keep the patient nonweight-bearing, ie, calcaneal osteotomy), and active inversion and eversion movements are encouraged. As an isolated procedure, PTT tendoscopy may be done as day surgery.

A posterior ankle arthroscopy approach may also be used for the treatment of PTT disorders. The use of a transflexor-hallucis-longus-tendon approach to penetrate the PTT sheath have been advocated with results comparable to those of conventional PTT tendoscopy and no neurovascular complications recorded.[16,18]

Posterior Tibial Tendon Tendoscopy: Findings and Treatment

Methodology for exploration and assessment of the PTT is fairly straightforward. Once the first portal is made, inversion of the foot may allow the arthroscope to advance

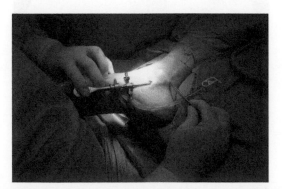

Fig. 4. Proximal portal is placed around 3 cm proximally to the tip of the medial malleolus.

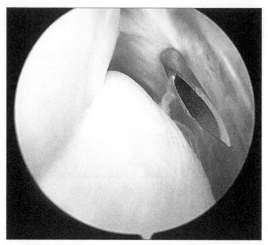

Fig. 5. Under direct visualization, a spinal needle is introduced to reference proximal portal.

easily and get a complete overview of the tendon to some 6–7 cm above the tip of the medial malleolus (**Fig. 7**). By rotating the scope, the complete tendon sheath can be inspected. The free edge of the vinculum can also be visualized and evaluated for abnormal thickening and debrided or resected if necessary (**Fig. 8**).

PTT adhesions and synovitis are the most common disorders encountered (**Fig. 9**). Adhesiolysis may be performed by using the probe to free the tendon from surrounding adhesions (Video 4). Synovectomy is usually carried out with a conventional shaver (**Fig. 10**) (Video 5). Partial ruptures can also be addressed (Video 6). Peripheral tears and frayed edges should be resected tendoscopically. Longitudinal tears may be reconstructed by tendon tubulization with the aid of a miniopen technique.

INDICATIONS FOR POSTERIOR TIBIAL TENDON TENDOSCOPY

Most indications for PTT open surgery are also indications for PTT tendoscopy.

There are many different scenarios that can cause PTT disorders.

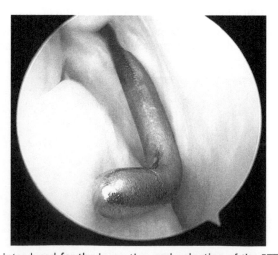

Fig. 6. A probe is introduced for the inspection and palpation of the PTT.

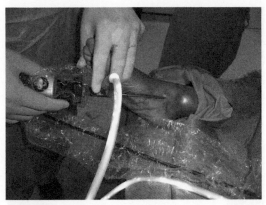

Fig. 7. Foot inversion allows for the scope to reach the vinculum, and the complete tendon is inspected.

Symptomatic Adult Flatfoot

Despite the strength of the tendon, an effective moment arm is required for the PTT to externally rotate the tibia and to supinate the foot. Excessive and continued pronation of the subtalar joint may render PTT insufficient. Tendinopathy may be followed by elongation and rupture. PTT dysfunction (PTTD) ranges from tenosynovitis to a rigid adult acquired flatfoot deformity.[19] Johnson and Strom classification was refined by Myerson.[20–22] Management of stages I and II involves dealing with PTT tendinopathy as part of the surgical strategy.

Stage I

Patients with stage I PTTD present with medial perimalleolar pain without foot deformity. Surgical debridement and synovectomy have been suggested when conservative measures do not achieve a pain-free ankle.[23] In cases of failed nonsurgical treatment of tenosynovitis or stenosis, or signs of tendon, degeneration surgical treatment with open synovectomy, tendon release and debridement provides good to

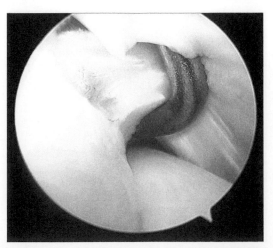

Fig. 8. The free edge of the vinculum is visualized and evaluated for abnormal thickening.

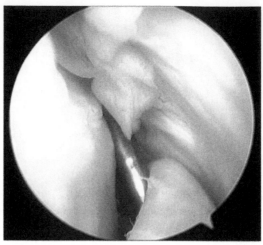

Fig. 9. PTT synovitis is a common finding in most patients undergoing this procedure.

excellent results (**Fig. 11**).[24] Tendoscopic debridement is also effective to improve function and pain in stage I PTTD. Chow and colleagues[25] and Khazen and colleagues[26] have advocated the use of tendoscopy for these patients with satisfactory results and less morbidity.

Stage II

Patients with stage II PTTD usually present with signs of tendinopathy and a flexible flatfoot deformity. Surgical treatment of stage II PTTD remains controversial.[27] Medial sliding calcaneal osteotomy seems to be the bony procedure of choice, with PTT debridement and flexor digitorum transfer being the soft tissue procedure to combine with osteotomy (**Fig. 12**). However, other tendon transfers have been proposed. Lui and colleagues[28] reported on anterior tibial tendon transfer and arthroereisis as a combined procedure. Endoscopic-assisted reconstruction of a torn PTT is advocated.

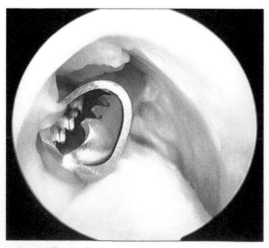

Fig. 10. Synovectomy is usually carried out with a shaver.

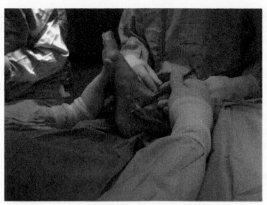

Fig. 11. Open debridement of PTT was the standard surgical procedure before tendoscopy came into practice.

Conventional portals are made to address the condition of PTT. Additional portals are made to gain access to anterior tibial tendon. The proximal portal is located at the musculotendinous junction of the anterior tibial tendon. The distal portal is located close to the anterior tibial tendon insertion, at the medial border of the dorsum of the foot. An anterior tibial tendoscopy is performed in order to harvest the medial half of the tendon while keeping the distal insertion intact. The diseased segment of PTT is excised, and the tendon graft is transferred. An augmentation by side-to-side suture with flexor digitorum longus through the PTT tendoscopy portals is recommended. These authors finally performed an arthroereisis with a bioabsorbable implant.[29]

Trauma

Direct or indirect trauma may be related to the development of tendinopathy and partial tears of the PTT. Blunt trauma over the medial malleolus may be responsible for pain and synovitis.

Typically, PTT rupture occurs in middle-aged and low sports active people,[30] but Woods and Leach reported on 6 athletes suffering from rupture.[31] Overuse disorders have been reported in different sports (dancers, ice-hockey) and its incidence is possibly underestimated.[32,33] Tenosynovitis has been reported in only 3% of active runners.[34]

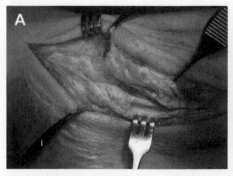
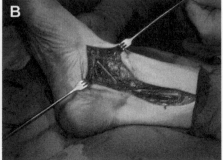

Fig. 12. (A) Conventional open debridement of a torn PTT. (B) Flexor digitorum transfer to PTT in stage II PTTD.

Irregularity of the posterior aspect of the tibia or incorrect screw placement following an ankle fracture may affect the sliding channel of the PTT and cause abnormal rubbing of the tendon. Postfracture adhesions may also alter normal movement of the tendon and cause synovitis and pain.

Dislocation/instability is quite uncommon when compared with peroneal tendon dislocation. It is usually found in athletes who have suffered repeated accidental injuries with inversion and dorsiflexion of the foot. Isolated anterior dislocation is the most rare PTT injury and has been documented only in terms of case reports, with special relation to ballet and running sports.[35–38] Tendoscopy may be useful to confirm dislocation and evaluate the extent of injury.

Systemic Inflammatory and Autoimmune Disorders

About half of the patients with rheumatoid arthritis could have PTTD.[39] Incidence of tendon synovitis and tears are high among patients with systemic inflammatory and autoimmune disorders (Video 7). The association of seronegative inflammatory disease and PTT tendinopathy has been well established. Younger patients apparently suffer from synovitis as a local manifestation of the systemic disease, whereas older patients suffer from the effects of mechanical trauma and degeneration.[40]

Iatrogenic Causes

Adhesions, scarring, and suboptimal medial malleolus screw placement may also induce tendinopathy (**Fig. 13**). Tendoscopy again is an option for the diagnosis and treatment of these disorders.

Except in the case of direct trauma, the development of PTT disease may progress from tendinopathy to elongation, degeneration, and rupture, and tendoscopy is a useful diagnostic and treatment tool in every stage.

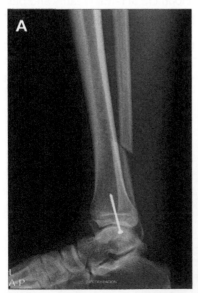
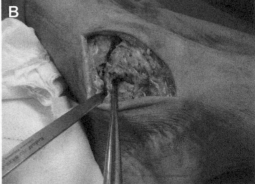

Fig. 13. (*A*) Suboptimal medial malleolus screw placement as part of an ankle fracture fixation. (*B*) Surgical treatment was needed to address medial malleolus nonunion and removal of screw that produced PTT synovitis.

There are some limitations for tendoscopy. Partial longitudinal tendon tears are difficult to be repaired endoscopically but new suture equipment will make it possible in the future.

DISCUSSION

PTT tendoscopy offers advantages over open procedures. There are fewer wound infections, less blood loss, smaller wounds, less morbidity, quicker recovery, early mobilization and function, mild postoperative pain, and the possibility of being performed under local anesthesia on an outpatient basis.

Advances in arthroscopic and endoscopic techniques have continued to expand indications for hindfoot tendoscopy. However, there are few quality evidence-based data in the current literature to support routine use of PTT tendoscopy. Only a few level IV and V studies are available on PTT tendoscopy. Several retrospective reviews have reported on the outcomes of PTT tendoscopy for a variety of indications. The diagnostic utility of this technique has become more widely recognized.

Van Dijk and colleagues[16] reported on the surgical technique and on the outcome of 16 patients with posteromedial pain on palpation over the PTT. Most patients were free of pain and showed no complications.

Bulstra and colleagues[41] published their experience with a series of 33 patients who underwent tendoscopy with good results for pathologic vincula and rheumatoid arthritis, but poor results for adhesiolysis, all with a low complication rate.

Chow and colleagues[25] reported on a series of 6 patients with synovectomy due to stage I PTTD with no complications and no progression to stage II PTTD.

Khazen and colleagues[26] performed PTT tendoscopies in 9 patients with stage I PTTD, with pain improvement in 8 patients.

Hua and colleagues[18] published a retrospective review of a series of 15 patients with PTT disorders with a posterior arthroscopic approach with no neurovascular complications and just one patient with a poor outcome.

Further research is needed in this area to have a more evidence-based approach to PTT disorders. Tendoscopy will possibly allow for a future classification of different findings in and around PTT. It will be important to establish which findings are physiologic or pathologic. Visualization of the tendon is only rivaled by open surgery, but with greater morbidity. To expand the use of this technique, new instrumentation dedicated for tendoscopy is required. The development of new endoscopic suture materials will allow for the treatment of longitudinal tears by means of tendoscopic tubulization, and new devices will possibly allow for the harvesting of flexor digitorum longus and transfer to the navicular. Meanwhile, PTT tendoscopy is probably nowadays the gold standard technique to diagnose and treat synovitis, small partial tears, adhesions, and stage I PTTD.

SUPPLEMENTARY DATA

Supplementary data related to this article can be found online at http://dx.doi.org/10.1016/j.fcl.2014.10.009.

REFERENCES

1. Kelikian AS, Sarrafian SK, Sarrafian SK. Sarrafian's anatomy of the foot and ankle: descriptive, topographical, functional. Philadelphia: Wolters Kluwer Health/ Lippincott Williams & Wilkins; 2011.
2. Lhoste-Trouilloud A. The tibialis posterior tendon. J Ultrasound 2012;15:2–6.

3. Petersen W, Hohmann G, Pufe T, et al. Structure of the human tibialis posterior tendon. Arch Orthop Trauma Surg 2004;124:237–42.
4. Benjamin M, Qin S, Ralphs JR. Fibrocartilage associated with human tendons and their pulleys. J Anat 1995;187:625–33.
5. Frey C, Shereff M, Greenidge N. Vascularity of the posterior tibial tendon. J Bone Joint Surg Am 1990;72A:884–8.
6. Petersen W, Hohmann G, Stein V, et al. The blood supply of the posterior tibial tendon. J Bone Joint Surg 2002;84B(1):141–4.
7. Prado MP, De Carvalho AE, Rodriguez CJ, et al. Vascular density of the posterior tibial tendon: a cadaver study. Foot Ankle Int 2006;27(8):628–31.
8. Roussignol X, Lagrave B, Berthiaux S, et al. Posterior tibial tendoscopy: description of an accessory proximal portal and assessment of tendon vascularization lesion according to portal. Foot Ankle Surg 2013;19(1):22–6.
9. Perry J, Schoneberger B. Gait analysis: normal and pathological function. Thorofare (NJ): Slack Inc; 1992.
10. Uchiyama E, Kitaoka HB, Fujii T, et al. Gliding resistance of the posterior tibial tendon. Foot Anke Int 2006;27(9):723–7.
11. Kaye RA, Jahss MH. Tibialis posterior: a review of anatomy and biomechanics in relation to support of the medial longitudinal arch. Foot Ankle 1991;11: 244–7.
12. Kong A, van der Vliet A. Imaging of tibialis posterior dysfunction. Br J Radiol 2008;81:826–36.
13. Rosenberg ZS, Cheung J, Jahss MH, et al. Rupture of posterior tibial tendon: CT and MR imaging with surgical correlation. Radiology 1988;169(1):229–35.
14. Schweitzer M, Karasick D. MR imaging of disorders of the posterior tibial tendon. Am J Roentgenol 2000;175:627–35.
15. Wertheimer SJ. The role of endoscopy in treatment of stenosing posterior tibial tenosynovitis. J Foot Ankle Surg 1995;34:15–22.
16. van Dijk CN, Knort N, Scholten PE. Tendoscopy of the posterior tibial tendon. Arthroscopy 1997;13(6):692–8.
17. Reilingh ML, de Leeuw PA, van Sterkenburg MN, et al. Tendoscopy of posterior tibial and peroneal tendons. Tech Foot Ankle Surg 2010;9(2):43–7.
18. Hua Y, Chen S, Li Y, et al. Arthroscopic treatment for posterior tibial tendon lesions with a posterior approach. Knee Surg Sports Traumatol Arthrosc 2013. [Epub ahead of print]. http://dx.doi.org/10.1007/s00167-013-2629-2.
19. van Sterkenburg MN, Haverkamp D, van Dijk CN, et al. A posterior tibial tendon skipping rope. Knee Surg Sports Traumatol Arthrosc 2010;18:1664–6.
20. Johnson KA, Strom DE. Tibialis posterior tendon dysfunction. Clin Orthop 1989; 179:275–83.
21. Johnson KA, Strom DE. Tibialis tendon dysfunction. Clin Orthop 1989;239: 196–206.
22. Bluman EM, Title CI, Myerson MS, et al. Posterior tibial tendon rupture: a refined classification system. Foot Ankle Clin 2007;8(3):637–45.
23. Bare AA, Haddad SL. Tenosynovitis of the posterior tibial tendon. Foot Ankle Clin 2001;6:37–66.
24. McCormack AP, Varner KE, Marymont JV. Surgical treatment for posterior tibial tendonitis in young competitive athletes. Foot Ankle Int 2003;24:535–8.
25. Chow HT, Chan KB, Lui TH. Tendoscopic debridement for stage I posterior tibial tendon dysfunction. Knee Surg Sports Traumatol Arthrosc 2005;13:695–8.
26. Khazen G, Khazen C. Tendoscopy in stage I posterior tibial tendon dysfunction. Foot Ankle Clin 2012;17(3):399–406.

27. Guha AR, Perera AM. Calcaneal osteotomy in the treatment of adult acquired flat-foot deformity. Foot Ankle Clin 2012;17(2):247–58.
28. Lui TH. Arthroscopy and endoscopy of the foot and ankle: indication for new techniques. Arthroscopy 2007;8:889–902.
29. Lui TH. Endoscopic assisted posterior tibial tendon reconstruction for stage 2 posterior tibial tendon insufficiency. Knee Surg Sports Traumatol Arthrosc 2007; 15(10):1228–34.
30. Holmes GB, Mann RA Jr. Possible epidemiological factors associated with rupture of the posterior tibial tendon. Foot Ankle 1992;13:70–9.
31. Woods L, Leach RE. Posterior tibial tendon rupture in athletic people. Am J Sports Med 1991;19:495–8.
32. Jacoby S, Slauterbeck J, Raikin S. Acute posterior tibial tendon tear in an ice-hockey player: a case report. Foot Ankle Int 2008;29(10):1045–8.
33. Angoules AG, Boutsikari EC. Posterior tibialis tendonitis in dancers. Clin Res Foot Ankle 2013;1:103.
34. Lysholm J, Wiklander J. Injuries in runners. Am J Sports Med 1987;15:168–71.
35. Larsen E, Lauridsen F. Dislocation of the tibialis posterior tendon in two athletes. Am J Sports Med 1984;12:429–30.
36. Ouzounian TJ, Myerson MS. Dislocation of the posterior tibial tendon. Foot Ankle 1992;13(4):215–9.
37. Khan KM, Gelber N, Slater K. Dislocated tibialis posterior tendon in a classical ballet dancer. J Dance Med Sci 1997;1:160–2.
38. Goucher NR, Coughlin MJ, Kristensen RM. Dislocation of the posterior tibial tendon: a literature review and presentation of two cases. Iowa Orthop J 2006; 26:122–6.
39. Michelson J, Easley M, Wigley FM, et al. Posterior tibial tendon dysfunction in rheumatoid arthritis. Foot Ankle Int 1995;16(3):156–61.
40. Myerson MS, Solomon G, Shereff M. Posterior tibial tendon dysfunction: its association with seronegative inflammatory disease. Foot Ankle 1989;9(5):219–25.
41. Bulstra GH, Olsthoom PG, van Dijk CN. Tendoscopy of the posterior tibial tendon. Foot Ankle Clin 2006;11(2):421–7.

Peroneal Tendoscopy

Tun Hing Lui, MBBS (HK), FRCS (Edin), FHKAM, FHKCOS[a],*,
Lung Fung Tse, FHKAM, FHKCOS[b]

KEYWORDS

- Peroneal tendoscopy • Retrofibular pain • Peroneal subluxation or dislocation
- Peroneal tendon tear • Tenosynovitis

KEY POINTS

- Peroneal tendoscopy was used primarily as a therapeutic procedure.
- It is seldom used simply for diagnosis purposes only.
- It is indicated for peroneal pathologies that failed conservative treatment.
- Peroneal tendoscopy offers dynamic assessment of tendon pathology.
- Endoscopic peroneal surgery is feasible for peroneal tenosynovitis, peroneal dislocation or subluxation, and partial tendon tear.

INTRODUCTION

Peroneal tendon abnormalities are responsible for most acute and chronic retrofibular ankle pain. Accurate clinical diagnosis of these disorders is often difficult and they are frequently underdiagnosed. Because arthroscopy of the ankle is now a well-established procedure used for diagnosis and treatment of foot and ankle disorders, peroneal tendoscopy could also be an effective tool for accurately diagnosing peroneal tendon abnormalities and treating some of these disorders.[1–4]

Peroneal tendon pathology can be categorized into three primary types: (1) tendinitis and tenosynovitis, (2) tendon subluxation and dislocation, and (3) tendon tears and ruptures. These conditions usually respond to nonoperative treatment. However, operative procedures of open debridement, tendon repair, and groove-deepening procedures are required in refractory cases.[2] With the advance of peroneal tendoscopy, peroneal tendon subluxation or dislocation can be dealt with by endoscopic superior peroneal retinaculum reconstruction[5] or endoscopic groove deepening.[6–8] Intrasheath dislocation can also be treated endoscopically.[9–11] Endoscopic resection of the peroneal tubercle (**Fig. 1**) can be performed if there is impingement to the peroneus longus tendon.[3,12] Endoscopic approaches have also been described to

The authors have nothing to disclose.
[a] Department of Orthopaedics and Traumatology, North District Hospital, 9 Po Kin Road, Sheung Shui, NT, Hong Kong 999077, China; [b] Department of Orthopaedics and Traumatology, Prince of Wales Hospital, Shatin, Hong Kong 999077, China
* Corresponding author.
E-mail address: luithderek@yahoo.co.uk

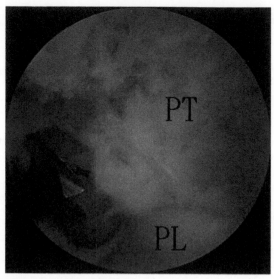

Fig. 1. Endoscopic resection of the peroneal tubercle. PL, peroneus longus tendon; PT, raw bone exposed after resection of the tubercle.

decompress the peroneal tendons in calcaneofibular impingement.[13,14] Endoscopic-assisted tendon repair is also performed in longitudinal tendon tears or complete tendon rupture.[15,16]

INDICATIONS

Indications for peroneal tendoscopy are shown in **Table 1**.

SURGICAL TECHNIQUE AND PROCEDURE
Preoperative Planning

1. Clinical assessment to confirm tenderness over the retrofibular region, the presence of synovitis, tendon thickening, or instability.
2. Medical imaging techniques including ultrasound and MRI are useful to detect underlying pathology causing peroneal abnormalities.
   a. Supernumerary or altered musculature in the lateral compartment of the leg.
   b. Accessory peroneus quartus (10%–26% of population),[21,22] peroneus digiti quinti, and peroneus accessorius muscles may be present and act as space-occupying lesions.[21,23] The peroneus brevis may be bifid, or normal muscle belly may extend too far distally (low-lying peroneal muscle belly) into the retromalleolar groove, causing an encroachment phenomenon.[24,25] The low-lying muscle bulk can be resected endoscopically if it causes symptoms (**Fig. 2**).[26]
   c. Both computed tomography and MRI are useful for detecting frankly subluxated or dislocated peroneal tendons by revealing the position of the tendons relative to the fibular groove.[27] The anatomic shape of the retromalleolar groove is evaluated on axial sections.

Patient Positioning

The patient can be positioned in lateral, anterior, or prone position for peroneal tendoscopy depending on any concomitant procedure that is planned to be performed. If

Table 1
Indications for peroneal tendoscopy

Indication	Author, Year of Publication	Outcome
Retrofibular pain	Lui,[15] 2012	6 of 7 patients (86%) resumed previous sport or activity within 24 mo
Snapping; diagnostic	van Dijk & Kort,[3] 1998	3 of 4 (75%) had no recurrence after adhesiolysis; 1 of 1 (100%) peroneal tubercle successfully removed; 1 of 1 (100%) longitudinal rupture successfully sutured
Tenosynovitis	Scholten & van Dijk,[17] 2006	10 chronic tenosynovitis have no recurrence of preoperative pathology
	Jerosch & Aldawoudy,[4] 2007	7 patients (100%) were symptom free at 3 mo postoperatively
Subluxation or dislocation	Guillo & Calder,[18] 2013	7 of 7 patients (100%) returned to previous activity level
	Vega et al,[19] 2013	Intrasheath subluxation: excellent results in 6 of 6 (100%; mean AOFAS score increased from 79 to 99)
Partial tears	Vega et al,[19] 2013	Ruptures, 15 of 24 (62.5%); symptom free, 6 of 24 (25%); partially symptom free, 3 of 24 (12.5%) no change
Postoperative adhesion and scarring, thickened vincula lesions	Marmotti et al,[20] 2012	5 of 5 patients (100%) reported subjective improvement of lateral ankle pain

Abbreviation: AOFAS, American Orthopaedic Foot & Ankle Society.

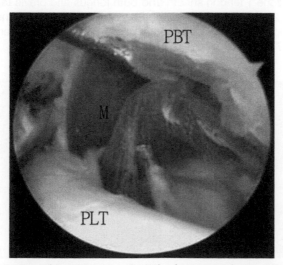

Fig. 2. Tendoscopic view of low lying muscle (M) of peroneus brevis. PBT, peroneus brevis tendon; PLT, peroneus longus tendon.

peroneal tendoscopy is the sole planned procedure, lateral position is preferred. A thigh tourniquet is applied to provide a bloodless surgical field.

Portal Design

1. Peroneal tendoscopy is performed with the proximal and distal portals along the course of the peroneal tendons. In general, proximal and distal portals are made 3 cm proximal and 1 cm distal to the lateral malleolar tip, respectively.
2. The locations of the portals should be made according to the exact location and extent of the pathology.
3. The working space of peroneal tendoscopy is limited by the boundary of the fibrous tendon sheath and the motion of the instruments allowed include in and out and rotation. Only a limited degree of side-to-side motion is allowed.
4. Coaxial portals are preferred because the portals are interchangeable as the visualization and working portals, and the whole span of the tendon sheath between the portals is reachable.
5. The commonly used tendoscopy portals cross the ankle joint and the peroneal tendon sheath is not a straight line when crossing this. The degree of passive ankle plantarflexion should be checked before making the portals because the tendon sheath is close to a straight line with ankle plantarflexion. If the degree of ankle plantarflexion is limited, the portals should be made closer to each other.
6. The proximal portals should be made more distally if the patient is obese or muscular. Otherwise, the mobility of the instruments through the proximal portal is hindered by the calf muscle or subcutaneous tissue.
7. The peroneal tendon sheaths are divided into three zones. The tendon sheath in zone 1 extends from the retrofibular groove to the peroneal tubercle. The peroneus longus and brevis tendons share a common tendon sheath in this zone. Zone 2 tendon sheath runs from the peroneal tubercle to the cuboid tunnel. The tendons have separate fibrous sheath at this zone. Zone 3 tendon sheath refers to the sheath of the peroneus longus tendon at the sole.[28]
8. The standard portals proximal and distal to the lateral malleolar tip are for assessment of the zone 1 tendon sheath and both longus and brevis tendon (**Fig. 3**).
9. During zone 2 tendoscopy, the longus and brevis tendon sheaths should be approached separately (**Fig. 4**). Because of the tightness of the tendon sheaths in this zone, 2.7-mm arthroscope is preferred.

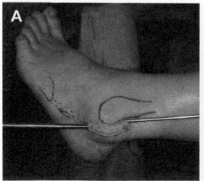 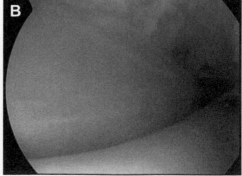

Fig. 3. (A) Zone 1 peroneal tendoscopy with portals proximal and distal to the lateral malleolar tip. (B) Arthroscopic view showed peroneus longus and brevis tendons.

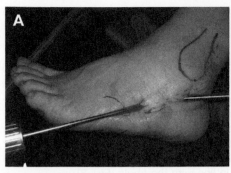
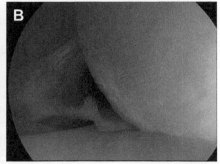

Fig. 4. (A) Zone 2 peroneal tendoscopy. (B) The tendons have their own tendon sheaths in this zone.

10. The tendon sheath for zone 3 can be approached through the plantar-lateral and plantar-medial portals (**Fig. 5**). The plantar-lateral portal is located distal to the turn of the peroneus longus tendon around the cuboid, which is 1 to 1.5 cm proximal and 1 cm plantar to the tip of the fifth metatarsal tubercle. The plantar-medial portal is at the plantar-lateral side of the base of the first metatarsal, which is close to the first tarsometatarsal joint. The portals should be identified with the aid of fluoroscopy. It should be noted that the portals of zone 3 tendon sheath are not interchangeable.
11. The portion of peroneus brevis tendon that is close to its insertion can be approached through the lateral Lisfranc portal, which is at the lateral corner of the fifth metatarsocuboid articulation.[29]

Surgical Procedure

1. After the portal sites are located, a 3- to 5-mm skin wound is made depending on the size of the arthroscope used. The subcutaneous tissue is bluntly dissected down to the tendon sheath by a hemostat and the tendon sheath is incised open.
2. A 2.7- or 4-mm 30-degree arthroscope is introduced via the distal portal.
3. Introduction of the instrument should be smooth and have no resistance. It should be done gently to avoid damage of the tendons.

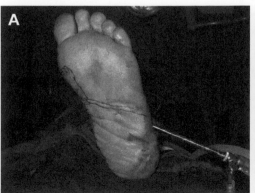
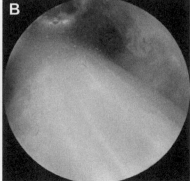

Fig. 5. (A) Zone 3 peroneal tendoscopy. (B) Only the peroneus longus tendon can be seen in this zone.

4. The peroneal tendons are examined for any tears or subluxation or dislocation. The superior peroneal retinaculum can be assessed for any tear or detachment from the fibula.
5. Endoscopic synovectomy is performed if tenosynovitis is present (**Fig. 6**).
6. Endoscopic groove deepening:
   a. The tendons are pushed medially by the arthroscope and the acromionizer if the tendon is not dislocatable.[12] In case of tendon instability, the tendons are dislocated anteriorly away from the retromalleolar groove and splinted by K wire.
   b. Endoscopic deepening of the retromalleolar groove is then performed with the acromionizer. We performed this procedure with the standard portals[15] rather than the three-portal approach.[7] We believe that this can create a smooth groove because the acromionizer is in line with the fibula (**Fig. 7**).
   c. The lateral cortical rim is left intact and the deepening procedure should extend to the most medial side of the groove. The deepening procedure should span from the most proximal end of distal fibular expansion down to the tip of the lateral malleolus.
   d. The posterior talofibular ligament and the posterior distal tibiofibular ligament should be preserved during the groove deepening.
7. Repair of longitudinal tear of the tendon:
   a. The exact location of the tear can be identified during the finger palpation along the tendons and can be visualized arthroscopically as dimpling of the superior peroneal retinaculum.
   b. Percutaneous suturing of the tendon tear can be performed with a curved eyed needle.
   c. The limbs of the suture are then retrieved to the portal wound under arthroscopic guide. Knotting can then be performed.
   d. In the case of an incomplete longitudinal tendon split, the limbs of suture should be retrieved at the same side of the tear to ensure that the knot is over the tear.
8. Superior peroneal retinaculum reconstruction:
   a. The distal portal is made just distal to lateral malleolar tip. The proximal portal is made at the proximal end of retinaculum, which is about 2 cm from the lateral malleolar tip.
   b. The tendons are pushed medially and splinted with K wires (**Fig. 8**).
   c. The lateral surface of lateral malleolus where retinaculum was stripped off is roughened with arthroscopic burr.

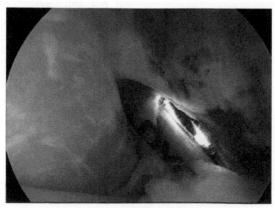

Fig. 6. Synovectomy of peroneal tendon sheath.

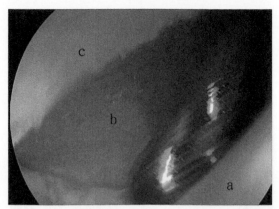

Fig. 7. Endoscopic retromalleolar groove deepening. (a) Peroneal tendon. (b) Deepened retromalleolar groove. (c) Lateral malleolus.

    d. Two to three suture anchors are inserted to the fibular ridge through the portals and are evenly spaced out along the span of elevated retinaculum (**Fig. 9**).

    e. The suture limbs are passed through the retinaculum by means of an eyed needle through the portals (**Fig. 10**). Sutures are retrieved at the surface of retinaculum to the portal wounds (**Fig. 11**).

    f. The retinaculum is pushed back to the bone manually and the sutures are tightened (**Fig. 12**).

COMPLICATIONS AND MANAGEMENT

Most complications are minor and include suture irritation. There is mild postoperative dyskinesia.[14] Most patients reported significant or complete relief of symptoms shortly after the procedure.

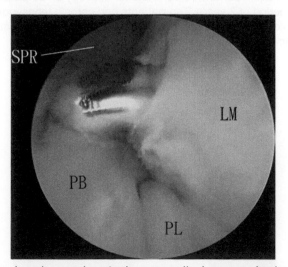

Fig. 8. The peroneal tendons are kept in the retromalleolar groove by the K wires that are inserted into the ridge of the retromalleolar groove. LM, lateral malleolus; PB, peroneus brevis tendon; PL, peroneus longus tendon; SPR, superior peroneal retinaculum.

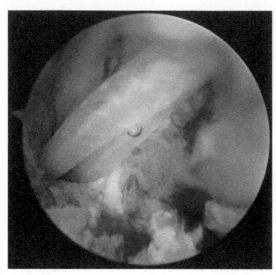

Fig. 9. Suture anchor is inserted in the ridge of the retromalleolar groove.

POSTOPERATIVE CARE

Postoperatively, ankle mobilization with inversion control ankle brace was advised. For those patients without tendon repair, early weight-bearing walking as pain tolerates is allowed. For those patients with tendon repair, non–weight bearing for 4 weeks is advised.

OUTCOME
Peroneal Tendinitis and Tenosynovitis

Scholten and van Dijk[17] performed peroneal tendoscopy on 23 patients with a minimum follow-up period of 2 years. Ten patients had chronic tenosynovitis and underwent tendoscopic synovectomy. None of the patients had complications, nor was there a recurrence of any preoperative pathology.

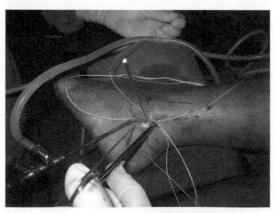

Fig. 10. The suture limbs passed through the retinaculum by means of an eyed needle through the portals.

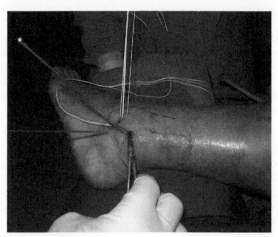

Fig. 11. Sutures are retrieved at the surface of retinaculum to the portal wounds.

Peroneal Subluxation and Dislocation and Peroneal Tendon Rupture

Vega and colleagues[19] reported a series of 52 patients who underwent peroneal tendoscopy from 2008 to 2011 with a minimum follow-up period of 1 year. The indications were peroneal adhesions (two), tenosynovitis (13), tendon rupture (24), recurrent peroneal tendon subluxation (seven), and intrasheath peroneal tendon subluxation (six). Of the 24 patients diagnosed with ruptures of the peroneal tendons, 15 (62.5%) reported complete relief of their symptoms, six (25%) reported partial relief, and three (12.5%) had no change in symptoms after the procedure. Of the seven patients treated with tendoscopic groove deepening for peroneal tendon subluxation, five (71.4%) reported excellent results and were able to return to their normal activities without limitations. No recurrent subluxation occurred at follow-up in any of the cases. All six patients treated for intrasheath subluxation had excellent results.

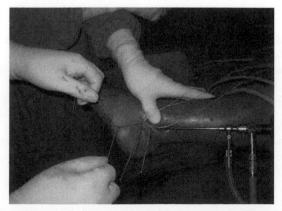

Fig. 12. The retinaculum is pushed back to the bone manually and the sutures are tightened.

SUMMARY

The peroneal tendoscopy technique has been gaining importance and popularity for the treatment of peroneal tendon pathologies. It allows anatomic evaluation of the tendons, and also provides dynamic assessment of the tendon position and mobility within the tendon sheaths through which the tendons move. Patients enjoyed the advantages of all minimally invasive surgeries, smaller scars, better cosmesis, less postoperative pain, shorter hospital stay, and higher patient satisfaction.

REFERENCES

1. Lui TH. Arthroscopy and endoscopy of the foot and ankle: indications for new techniques. Arthroscopy 2007;23:889–902.
2. Heckman DS, Reddy S, Pedowitz D, et al. Current concepts review: operative treatment for peroneal tendon disorders. J Bone Joint Surg Am 2008;90:404–18.
3. Dijk van CN, Kort N. Tendoscopy of the peroneal tendons. Arthroscopy 1998;14: 471–8.
4. Jerosch J, Aldawoudy A. Tendoscopic management of peroneal tendon disorders. Knee Surg Sports Traumatol Arthrosc 2007;15:806–10.
5. Lui TH. Endoscopic peroneal retinaculum reconstruction. Knee Surg Sports Traumatol Arthrosc 2006;14:478–81.
6. Title CI, Jung HG, Parks BG, et al. The peroneal groove deepening procedure: a biomechanical study of pressure reduction. Foot Ankle Int 2005;26:442–8.
7. de Leeuw PA, van Dijk CN, Golanó P. A 3-portal endoscopic groove deepening technique for recurrent peroneal tendon dislocation. Tech Foot Ankle Surg 2008;7:250–6.
8. Porter D, McCarroll J, Knapp E, et al. Peroneal tendon subluxation in athletes: fibular groove deepening and retinacular reconstruction. Foot Ankle Int 2005; 26:436–41.
9. Raikin SM, Elias I, Nazarian LN. Intrasheath subluxation of the peroneal tendons. J Bone Joint Surg Am 2008;90:992–9.
10. Thomas JL, Lopez-Ben R, Maddox J. A preliminary report on intrasheath peroneal tendon subluxation: a prospective review of 7 patients with ultrasound verification. J Foot Ankle Surg 2009;48:323–9.
11. Michels F, Jambou S, Guillo S, et al. Endoscopic treatment of intrasheath peroneal tendon subluxation. Case Rep Med 2013;2013:274685.
12. Lui TH. Endoscopic resection of the peroneal tubercle. J Foot Ankle Surg 2012; 51:813–5.
13. Bauer T, Deranlot J, Hardy P. Endoscopic treatment of calcaneo-fibular impingement. Knee Surg Sports Traumatol Arthrosc 2011;19:131–6.
14. Lui TH. Endoscopic lateral calcaneal ostectomy for calcaneofibular impingement. Arch Orthop Trauma Surg 2007;127:265–7.
15. Lui TH. Endoscopic management of recalcitrant retrofibular pain without peroneal tendon subluxation or dislocation. Arch Orthop Trauma Surg 2012;132: 357–61.
16. Ho KK, Chan KB, Lui TH, et al. Tendoscopic-assisted repair of complete rupture of the peroneus longus associated with displaced fracture of the os peroneum: case report. Foot Ankle Int 2013;34:1600–4.
17. Scholten PE, van Dijk CN. Tendoscopy of the peroneal tendons. Foot Ankle Clin 2006;11:415–20.
18. Guillo S, Calder JDF. Treatment of recurring peroneal tendon subluxation in athletes. Endoscopic repair of the retinaculum. Foot Ankle Clin 2013;18:293–300.

19. Vega J, Golanó P, Batista JP, et al. Tendoscopic procedure associated with peroneal tendons. Tech Foot Ankle Surg 2013;12:39–48.
20. Marmotti A, Cravino M, Germano M, et al. Peroneal tendoscopy. Curr Rev Musculoskelet Med 2012;5:135–44.
21. Cheung YY, Rosenberg ZS, Ramsinghani R, et al. Peroneus quartus muscle: MR imaging features. Radiology 1997;202:745.
22. Hutchimon BL, Gustafson LS. Chronic peroneal tendon subluxation: new surgical technique and retrospective analysis. J Am Podiatr Med Assoc 1994;84:511–7.
23. Butler BW, Lanthier J, Wertheimer SJ. Subluxing peroneals: a review of the literature and case report. J Foot Ankle Surg 1993;32:134–9.
24. Sammarco GJ, Brainard BJ. A symptomatic anomalous peroneus brevis in a high-jumper. J Bone Joint Surg Am 1991;73:131.
25. Clarke HD, Kitaoka HB, Ehman RL. Peroneal tendon injuries. Foot Ankle Int 1998;19:280–8.
26. Lui TH. Tendoscopic resection of low-lying muscle belly of peroneus brevis or quartus. Foot Ankle Int 2012;33:912–4.
27. Mota J, Rosenberg ZS. Magnetic resonance imaging of the peroneal tendons. Top Magn Reson Imaging 1998;9:273–85.
28. Lui TH. Tendoscopy of peroneus longus in the sole. Foot Ankle Int 2013;34:299–302.
29. Lui TH. Lateral foot pain following open reduction and internal fixation of the fracture of the fifth metatarsal tubercle: treated by arthroscopic arthrolysis and endoscopic tenolysis. BMJ Case Rep 2014;2014.

Achilles Tendoscopy

Dominic Carreira, MD[a],*, Alicia Ballard, DO[b]

KEYWORDS

- Achilles tendoscopy • Achilles tendinopathy • Equinus contracture • Achilles rupture
- Haglund's deformity • Noninsertional Achilles tendinopathy

KEY POINTS

- The Achilles tendon is technically accessible through an endoscopic approach because of its location in a well-formed tunnel.
- Minimally invasive treatment of equinus contracture, Achilles rupture, Haglund's deformity, and other less proven pathologies are also discussed yields good clinical results.
- A thorough understanding of the surgical anatomy and endoscopic technique minimizes complications.

Videos of endoscopic gastrocnemius release and endoscopic treatment for Haglund's deformity accompany this article at http://www.foot.theclinics.com/

INTRODUCTION

Endoscopic surgery provides a minimally invasive approach to visualize and treat several pathologic conditions of the Achilles tendon. In comparision with endoscopic surgeries, open surgery of the hindfoot has been associated with wound complications, whereas endoscopic procedures have been recognized for less scarring, less perioperative pain, fewer wound complications, and faster recovery.[1] Various endoscopic techniques have been described for the treatment of pathologies related to the Achilles, including equinus contracture, Achilles rupture, Haglund's deformity, and noninsertional Achilles tendinopathy.

ANATOMY

The Achilles tendon is the strongest and thickest tendon in the human body.[1] It measures on average 12 cm to 15 cm long and is the confluence of the aponeuroses of the

A. Ballard, DO has identified no professional or financial affiliations with themselves or spouse/partner; D. Carreira, MD is a paid consultant for Biomet Sports Medicine.

[a] Orthopedics and Sports Medicine, Broward Health, NOVA Southeastern University, 300 Southeast 17th Street, Fort Lauderdale, FL 33316, USA; [b] Orthopedic Department, Broward Health, 1600 South Andrews Avenue, Fort Lauderdale, FL 33316, USA
* Corresponding author.
E-mail address: Dcarreira@browardhealth.org

Foot Ankle Clin N Am 20 (2015) 27–40
http://dx.doi.org/10.1016/j.fcl.2014.10.003
1083-7515/15/$ – see front matter © 2015 Elsevier Inc. All rights reserved.

soleus and gastrocnemius muscles. Both muscles are innervated by the tibial nerve and together make up the triceps surae. The gastrocnemius muscle unit is made up of the medial and lateral heads, and originates off the distal femur. The muscle crosses the knee, ankle, and subtalar joints before inserting into the calcaneus. The soleus muscle originates off of the proximal tibia and fibula posteriorly and crosses only the ankle and subtalar joints before its insertion. The Achilles tendon inserts into the calcaneus approximately 13 mm below the most proximal aspect of the calcaneus tuberosity.[2] Proximally, the gastrocnemius is posterior to the soleus muscle; however, it undergoes a 90° twist so that the gastrocnemius inserts into the lateral aspect of the posterior calcaneus, whereas the soleus inserts along the medial aspect of the posterior calcaneus.

The Achilles tendon is surrounded by a paratenon and does not have a tendon sheath. The paratenon is separated into an inner visceral and outer parietal layer with an interposing mesotenon layer, the site for the blood supply. At the site of insertion, the Achilles tendon receives a limited blood supply from periosteal and osseus vessels. For this reason, degenerative changes are often seen in this area. In the space between the ventral side of the Achilles tendon and the calcaneus lies the retrocalcaneal bursa. Kager's triangle is a fat pad that sits anterior to the Achilles tendon and can be detected on the lateral radiograph. The triangle is disturbed by chronic inflammation of the bursa, which can occasionally be detected on plain films.[1,3]

BIOMECHANICS

The Achilles tendon sustains up to 12.5 times of body weight during certain running activities, and the gastrocnemius and soleus muscles account for approximately 90% of energy in plantarflexion.[4,5] During the gait cycle, maximum tension is placed on the tendon in late-stance phase. When the knee is in extension, the gastrocnemius tendon limits the degree of dorsiflexion, whereas the entire triceps surae can limit dorsiflexion with the knee in flexion. Late-stance phase dorsiflexion beyond 10° is dependent on the flexibility of the gastrocnemius muscle unit.[6,7]

EQUINUS CONTRACTURE

Heel cord tightness has been linked to multiple pathologic conditions, including metatarsalgia, Morton's neuroma, flatfoot deformity, and plantar fasciitis.[8] Heel cord tightness is commonly associated with spastic neurologic deformities, such as cerebral palsy, or with congenital deformities, such as clubfoot,[6] but it is most commonly noted in patients without preexisting deformity who are neurologically normal. An equinus contracture increases peak plantar pressure and can lead to the development of plantar foot ulcers in patients with neuropathy, especially in diabetics.[9] Furthermore, as a compensatory adaptation during the gait cycle, the biomechanics of the late-stance phase may be altered with an equinus contracture, and patients may externally rotate to facilitate rolling over the forefoot.[10]

Criterion for an isolated gastrocnemius contracture is defined as ≤5°of maximal ankle dorsiflexion with the knee in full extension. A triceps surae contracture is defined as ≤10° dorsiflexion with the knee in 90° of flexion.[6] A positive Silfverskiöld maneuver indicates passive dorsiflexion beyond neutral with the knee flexed but limited dorsiflexion with the knee extended and differentiates an isolated gastrocnemius contracture.[11]

Historically, the most frequently used surgical treatments for equinus contractures have been open gastrocnemius releases or percutaneous Achilles tenotomy.[8] With the open gastrocnemius approach, wound healing, unsightly incisions, tethering of the skin to the underlying fascia, and sural nerve irritation have been cited as reasons for patient dissatisfaction.[12] Percutaneous tenotomy has been associated with excessive release, thereby effectively overlengthening the Achilles, with resulting pain from calcaneal gait pattern.[13,14] With the endoscopic approach for gastrocnemius release, decreased morbidity and faster recovery times have been noted.[15]

Indications for Endoscopic Gastrocnemius Release

- Loss of ankle dorsiflexion causing pain and/or altered gait
- Protracted forefoot/midfoot pain with 0° or less of ankle dorsiflexion when the knee is in full extension[10]
- Diabetic forefoot ulcer with 5° or less of ankle dorsiflexion with the knee in full extension
- Contracture causing heel valgus and flatfoot alignment during the gait cycle
- Knee pain resulting from compensatory hyperextension at the knee joint
- Decreased vascularity, diabetes, or compromised skin or other condition in which the host is compromised (in association with the indications noted above)

Technique

The patient is placed on the operating table in the supine or prone position with a pneumatic tourniquet placed on the thigh and inflated. The choice of patient positioning is most dependent on other associated procedures performed at the time of surgery but is preferably the prone position. The musculotendinous junction of the gastrocnemius is identified. Correct medial portal placement is crucial to performing an isolated gastrocnemius release and to avoiding damage to the sural nerve (**Fig. 1**).

Cadaveric anatomic studies have found that on the medial side of the calf, the proximal extent of the gastrocnemius tendon is located between 38% and 46% of the distance between the fibular head and the upper border of the calcaneus.[16] Several guidelines have been reported for placement of the medial portal (**Box 1**).

The senior author places the medial portal one inch distal to the palpable musculotendinous junction (**Fig. 2**). Ultrasound confirmation of the musculotendinous junction may be used in patients whose anatomy is difficult to palpate.

An arthroscopic switching stick is inserted through the medial portal in the plane between the deep fascia and the posterior gastrocnemius to increase the working space with a sweeping motion. Several commercially available endoscopic carpal tunnel systems are available that provide a slotted cannula through which the gastrocnemius tendon can be endoscopically visualized and through which a retrograde cutting knife can be safely passed. The lateral portal is established with an inside-out technique, and a nick and spread technique is used to protect the sural nerve. A 4-mm scope is inserted medially as part of a dry endoscopic technique. The gastrocnemius tendon is a brighter white color and has tightly packed parallel fibers compared with the more superficial posterior fascia. To maintain a dry field, a cotton tipped probe may be placed laterally or, alternatively, the slotted cannula can be pushed out laterally and into the tip of a Yankauer suction tip. The posterior aspect of the gastrocnemius tendon is visualized, and care is taken to ensure that the sural nerve is not in the plane anterior to the cannula. The retrograde knife is introduced from the lateral portal and the ankle is held in dorsiflexion. The gastrocnemius tendon is released medial to lateral. Slow and careful recession on the lateral side is recommended to ensure that the sural nerve is preserved. Medially, the tendon curves anteriorly and may need additional release (**Fig. 3**). The endoscopic system can then be removed, and the camera can be introduced to check the extent of release while maintaining the same position of ankle dorsiflexion so as to maintain visualization of the area of recession. A complete release should allow the ankle to dorsiflex to at least 10° with the knee extended. An additional

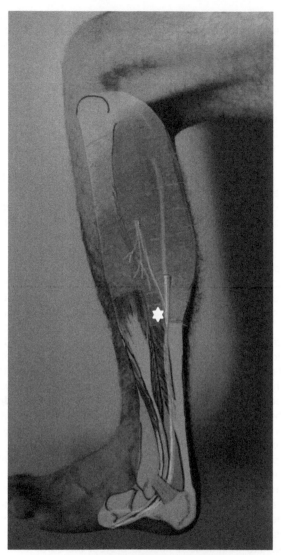

Fig. 1. Lateral diagram shows the proximity of the sural nerve to the location of the lateral portal, one inch distal to musculoskeletal junction. Portal location marked with a star.

percutaneous Achilles tenotomy may also be considered in patients with higher degrees of contracture in whom contracture persists (Video 1).

The patient is placed in a boot and allowed to bear weight immediately with the use of crutches as needed. Patients are instructed to begin range of motion exercises after the first dressing change. Sutures are removed in 7 to 10 days. After 4 to 6 weeks, patients are weaned from the boot.

Results

Both 1-portal and 2-portal techniques have been described, both with satisfactory outcomes.[10,15] On average, an equinus contracture was improved by 12° to 18° toward dorsiflexion with a dual portal technique.[10] Tashjian performed this technique

Box 1
Anatomic descriptions of medial portal placement for endoscopic gastrocnemius release for equinus contracture

Medial Portal Placement

2 cm distal to the visible indent of the musculotendinous junction[17,18]

Four finger breadths proximal to the flare of medial malleolus[19]

Distal to the junction of the middle and distal thirds of the leg[20]

16 to 17 cm proximal to the distal tip of the medial malleolus[21]

16.40 cm proximal to the calcaneus[22]

At 50% of the fibula's length proximal to its distal tip[23]

on cadaver models and reported an incomplete release in 17% because of the curve of the tendon anteriorly on both sides but reported an immediate gain of 20° of dorsiflexion.[17] Mini-open incisions were recommended on both sides to identify the borders. Grady and Kelly[24] reported on 23 healthy pediatric and adolescent patients who underwent 40 procedures with the 2-portal technique. Dorsiflexion improved by a mean of 15°, and no patient reported diminished nerve sensation postoperatively.

Roukis and Schweinberger reported a complication rate of 11.3% (3 of 21 patients) in patients treated with a single portal approach for spastic contracture. These patients were reported to have undercorrection of the ankle equinus deformity.[25] They concluded that this was owing to patient selection. Saxena and Widfeldt[26] performed a prospective, multisurgeon, multicenter analysis of the uniportal endoscopic gastrocnemius recession in 47 patients (54 procedures). Dorsiflexion improved significantly from -8° ± 4° to 7° ± 4° postoperatively. Lateral dysesthesia (11%) and unacceptable cosmesis (11%) were the most common complications reported. Weakness in plantarflexion was reported but found to be temporary. Saxena and Widfeldt[27] reported return of single leg raise function 13 weeks after endoscopic gastrocnemius recession. Tashjian reported sural nerve laceration in one specimen in his cadaver study, and sural nerve dysesthesias were reported in up to 15% of patients.[23] This complication was thought to be caused by direct injury or from tendon lengthening.

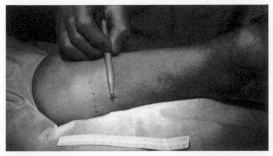

Fig. 2. Medial portal placement for gastrocnemius release, 1 inch distal to the palpable musculoskeletal junction.

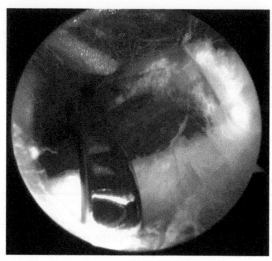

Fig. 3. Intraoperative view of gastrocnemius after release.

ACHILLES RUPTURE

The incidence of Achilles ruptures is trending upward along with the popularity of recreational sporting activities.[28,29] Although some controversy exists related to the operative versus nonoperative treatment of Achilles ruptures, operative over nonoperative treatment has shown a decreased rerupture rate, stronger push off, less calf atrophy, and earlier functional treatment.[30–32] Because the main complication of open surgery has been wound problems including infection,[28] percutaneous, mini-open, and endoscopic techniques are described as alternatives to the open approach.

Ma and Griffith[33] described an entirely percutaneous approach with very good results. Subsequent reports, however, have reported a higher complication rate including sural nerve injury, stump misalignment, decreased strength at the rupture site, and increased rate of rerupture.[34] A minimally invasive approach using approximately 2 cm incisions and a jig has demonstrated excellent results and gained popularity in recent years. In this approach, the jig allows the surgeon to identify the tendon within the paratenon and thereby pass suture without capturing the sural nerve. This technique is the preferred technique by the senior author. Here we also present an all-endsocopic technique and published outcomes.

Proposed advantages of an endoscopically assisted percutaneous repair include evaluation of the tendon quality, debridement and mobilization of the tendon ends, accurate passage of needles, and guided approximation of the tendon ends.[10,35,36] Few surgeons have adopted this technique, citing concerns with limited visualization of both the tendon and the sural nerve.

Indications

- Acute midsubstance Achilles tendon ruptures within 10 days of injury[10]

Technique

The patient is placed in a prone position and a pneumatic tourniquet is applied to the thigh. The unaffected ankle is examined with the knee in flexion to gauge the amount of resting plantarflexion. The tendon gap is outlined on the operative leg. A modified Ma-Griffith technique as described by Halasi[36] is used to create a 4-strand construct.[10] Six portals are used, as described by Ma and Griffith.[33] One portal is placed on each side of the tendon, at the proximal and distal and at the level of the tear. An arthroscopic cannula is placed at the medial-distal portal into the tendon gap, and the tear is inspected as the paratenon sheath is inflated with fluid on low pressure. The hematoma is evacuated, and the tendon ends are debrided if necessary. Number 2 suture is used in a double suture configuration. The needle is first introduced through the medial-proximal portal through the tendon, and out transversely through the lateral-proximal portal. To avoid sural nerve damage, a soft tissue protector, such as a drill guide, is used at the proximal lateral incision. The protector is placed on the paratenon through the subcutaneous tissues, and a straight needle is guided through the first transverse step of suture.[36] The protector is not moved after this step, only angled 60° distal so that the sural nerve remains protected from suturing. After the construct with the 2 suture loops is created, the ankle is held in plantarflexion and the sutures are tied, ensuring the appropriate tension on the tendon when compared with the opposite side. The patient is immobilized in a splint for 3 weeks and started in early functional rehabilitation in a boot with a heel lift for an additional 5 weeks.[36]

Results

Halasi and colleagues[36] reported improved rerupture rate and comparable strength, calf atrophy, and return to activities when he compared endoscopic-assisted percutaneous repair versus percutaneous repair alone. The lower rerupture rate was attributed to the ability to better control the tendon ends with direct visualization with the endoscope. Turgut and colleagues[35] reported on 11 patients treated with the endoscopic assisted Ma-Griffith approach. There were no reruptures, wound problems, or neurovascular injuries reported. Tang treated 20 patients with endoscopically assisted Kessler's technique and reported excellent results in 15 cases and good results in 5 cases using the Lindholm scale. No complications were reported.[37] Fortls and colleagues[34] found 12% decrease in maximum torque and 16.5% decrease in work performance on the injured side in 20 patients treated with the Ma-Griffith technique. Sural neuralgia was reported in 2 patients, one of which resolved without further intervention.[34] An endoscopic-assisted percutaneous repair with a modified Bunnell was performed by Doral and colleagues[38] in 62 patients with 100% satisfactory results and a mean American Orthopaedic Foot & Ankle Society score of 94.6. Two patients reported a transient sural nerve hypoesthesia that resolved after 6 months, and 95% of patients returned to their previous sport activities. In the setting of chronic noninsertional Achilles ruptures, case reports of endoscopic-assisted repair with flexor hallucis tendon transfer have been described with promising results.[39,40]

HAGLUND'S SYNDROME

The posterosuperior aspect of the os calcis may be enlarged and painful, with or without Achilles tendinopathy and retrocalcaneal bursitis. The condition, known as a Haglund's deformity or "pump bump," has long been associated with a rigid heel counter (**Fig. 4**).[41,42] Nonoperative treatment consists of eccentric strengthening of the Achilles, shoe wear modifications, nonsteroidal anti-inflammatory drugs, night splinting, heel inserts, rest, and immobilization. However, 50% to 65% of patients do not respond to nonsurgical measures after 6 months.[42]

The traditional operative approach includes open debridement of the tendon, retrocalcaneal bursectomy, and resection of the posterosuperior aspect of the calcaneus.[43] Depending on the extent of Achilles takedown and debridement, the Achilles may be reattached. Rare complications described with this open technique

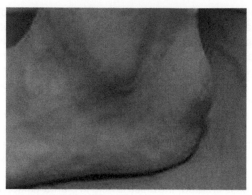

Fig. 4. Clinical picture of Haglund's deformity.

include skin breakdown, Achilles avulsion, scar hypersensitivity, altered skin sensation about the heel, inadequate resection, and postoperative stiffness.[44] Because Achilles insertional tendinopathy is typically extensive in these patients with Haglund's disease, the open approach with concomitant debridement and fixation is most commonly performed. Painful nodules along the Achilles tendon indicate noninsertional Achilles tendinopathy for which endoscopic calcaneoplasty is not indicated.[43] The endoscopic approach may be used, particularly in younger patients who have little to no Achilles tendinopathy. The first series of endoscopic calcaneoplasties for Haglund's syndrome was reported by van Dijk and colleagues[45] in 2001, and others have also reported success.[10,43,45] Appropriate preoperative workup is necessary for more predictable results. On physical examination, the ideal patient has tenderness to palpation on the superolateral aspect of the calcaneus.[10] MRI can be useful to rule out intrasubstance tendon degeneration. A lateral radiograph of the hindfoot is necessary to evaluate the posterosuperior calcaneal border, the presence of calcaneal spurring at the insertion of the tendon, and obliteration of Kager's triangle caused by the presence of retrocalcaneal bursitis.[46]

Indications

- Painful enlarged posterosuperior border of the os calcis with or without recalcitrant retrocalcaneal bursitis[10]

Technique

The patient is placed prone or supine on the operating table with a pneumatic tourniquet on the thigh (**Fig. 5**). The lateral portal is made through a vertical incision at the level of the superior aspect of the calcaneus (**Fig. 6**). The incision is made immediately adjacent to the Achilles tendon (slightly anterior and lateral) and is carried down bluntly to minimize the risk to the sural nerve branch. The retrocalcaneal space is entered with a blunt trochar. A 4.0-mm scope is placed, and a medial portal is similarly established using the light of the arthroscope. The bursal tissue is removed with a 4.0-mm shaver introduced through the medial portal. The Achilles attachment and posterior calcaneus can now be inspected. The posterosuperior calcaneal prominence is resected with the 4.0 arthroscopic hooded burr, ensuring that the tendon is protected. Adequacy of the excision is confirmed by absence of posterior impingement with the ankle in full dorsiflexion and with lateral fluoroscopy images. Damage to the Achilles tendon can be removed with the shaver. In the setting of limited areas of chronically degenerated tendon, an 18-gauge needle can be used to trephinate these sections to initiate

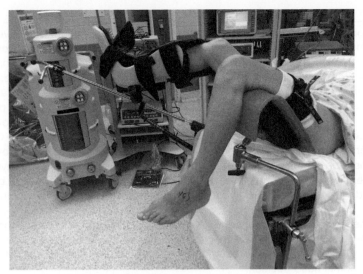

Fig. 5. Supine positioning for endoscopic calcaneoplasty, the senior author's preferred position. The operative leg is held with a posterior thigh pad, whereas the contralateral leg is held abducted in a gynecology leg positioner.

a vascular response.[44] The patient is instructed to remain non–weight bearing for 2 weeks followed by range-of-motion exercises and weight bearing in a boot for the subsequent 2 weeks. Return to normal footwear may be initiated as early as 4 weeks (Video 2).

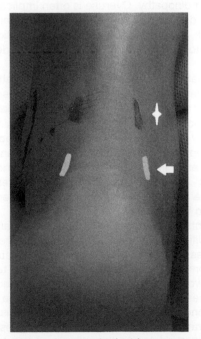

Fig. 6. Portal locations for calcaneoplasty marked with arrow. Standard portals for hindfoot tendoscopy indicated with star.

Results

Endoscopic calcaneoplasty has been successful in treating patients who have a painful prominence of the posterosuperior aspect of the calcaneus with retrocalcaneal bursitis.[10,43,45] In van Dijk and colleagues[45] initial series of 20 patients, 19 had good to excellent results with return to sport after 12 weeks. Jerosch and colleagues[47] studied 81 patients for an average of 35.3 months after endoscopic calcaneoplasty. The Ogilvie-Harris score was excellent in 41 patients, good in 34, fair in 3, and poor in 3 patients.[47] The patients with poor results were revised with an open approach and it was found that these patients had ossification of the Achilles tendon. Ortmann and McBryd[44] reported on 28 patients (30 heels) with an average follow-up of 35 months. The American Orthopaedic Foot & Ankle Society score improved from 62 preoperatively to 97 postoperatively. There were 26 excellent results, 3 good results, and 1 poor result. No wound complications or postoperative infections occurred, but Achilles tendon rupture 3 weeks after surgery and residual pain and swelling necessitated open procedure in 2 patients. Labib and Pendleton[43] described an "improved technique" in which the patient is prone with the surgeon standing at the ipsilateral side of the ankle with the monitor at the end of the table, which allowed a more ergonomic hand position.

NONINSERTIONAL ACHILLES TENDINOPATHY

Noninsertional pathology of the Achilles tendon is a common condition among runners and athletes and can occur acutely or chronically. It can be classified as tendinopathy, paratendinopathy, or as a combination of the 2. Symptoms include painful swelling of the Achilles tendon, typically 4 cm to 6 cm proximal to its insertion.[1] The swelling moves up and down with passive dorsiflexion and plantarflexion in tendinopathy but does not move in paratendinopathy. Overuse is often implicated in this disorder, but other factors have been described. Misalignment, poor training technique, improper training surface, strength imbalance, compression and friction of the tendon, shoe-related factors, rheumatoid arthritis, and endocrine disorders may predispose to this condition.[48]

Patients with tendinopathy can present with 3 different patterns: diffuse thickening of the tendon, local degeneration of the tendon but mechanically intact, or insufficiency of the tendon with rupture. Patients with paratendinopathy have a notable painful swelling of the paratenon, and only the paratenon is involved on MRI. Patients with chronic paratendinopathy often complain of pain on the medial side.[49] Medially, the soleus and plantaris tendons are separated by the paratenon. Simultaneous knee and ankle movements result in a different pull of both tendons at the same level because of the muscles' different origins. In a healthy patient, the plantaris tendon can glide in relation to the Achilles tendon; however, in paratendinopathy the plantaris tendon becomes fixed to the Achilles tendon.[1]

Conservative treatments consist of nonsteroidal anti-inflammatory drugs, activity modifications, shoe modifications, shoe inserts, eccentric stretching, and immobilization.[1,10] If the patient does not respond to conservative measures after 6 months, surgical intervention is recommended. Standard open Achilles tendon debridement has been associated with wound complications, prolonged recovery, and scarring.[50] Endoscopic treatment has been successfully applied to the goals of open surgery: decompression of the tendon by excision of degenerative tissue, lysis of adhesions, excision of thickened paratenon, and stimulation of healing response.[1] No clear guidelines have been established related to the efficacy of this technique related to the extent of tendon degeneration.

Indication

- Noninsertional Achilles tendinopathy with failure of appropriate nonsurgical treatment[10]

Technique

As described by van Dijk and colleagues,[45] the patient is placed prone on the operating table and a pneumatic tourniquet is placed on the thigh. The foot must be at the end of the table to allow the surgeon to move the foot in full dorsiflexion and plantarflexion. The distal portal is located on the lateral border of the Achilles tendon 2 to 3 cm distal to the pathologic thickening. The proximal portal is located 2 to 4 cm proximal to the thickening. This arrangement allows for approximately 10 cm of length to visualize and work along the Achilles tendon. The lateral portal is placed first. A small skin incision is made, followed by blunt dissection with a 2.7-mm trochar in a proximal direction. The trochar can be used to release any adhesions in the paratenon space by passing it around the tendon. The 30° 2.7-mm arthroscope is introduced and gravity inflow is used for insufflation. Under direct visualization, a spinal needle is introduced proximally for localization of a second portal.

Any fibrotic tissue binding the tendon to the sheath can be removed under direct visualization with a full radius shaver. The plantaris tendon can now be identified just medial to the Achilles tendon and, in the case of paratendinopathy, can be released. Resection of the paratenon is performed on the anterior side of the tendon at the level of the painful nodule.

The patient is allowed to bear weight as tolerated, and is instructed to keep the foot elevated when not ambulatory. Active range-of-motion exercises are encouraged.

Results

Steenstra and van Dijik[1] successfully treated 20 patients with noninsertional tendinopathy without complications. The Foot and Ankle Outcome and SF-6 scores at average of 6 years were comparable to those in a cohort of people without Achilles tendon complaints. Lui[51] also described an endoscopic Achilles tendon debridement with flexor hallucis longus transfer in 5 patients with chronic noninsertional Achilles tendinopathy with good results. Maquirriain[52] performed endoscopic debridement of peritendinous tissue with percutaneous longitudinal tenotomies when tendinopathy was present. Complete resolution of symptoms at 7 years postoperatively was seen in 96% of the patients.

SUMMARY

The Achilles tendon is technically accessible through an endoscopic approach because of its location in a well-formed tunnel. Minimally invasive treatment of equinus contracture, Achilles rupture, Haglund's deformity, and noninsertional Achilles tendinopathy yield good clinical results, and the technique has the advantages that are related to any minimally invasive procedure. A thorough understanding of the surgical anatomy and endoscopic technique minimizes complications.

SUPPLEMENTARY DATA

Supplementary data accompany this article at http://dx.doi.org/10.1016/j.fcl.2014. 10.003.

REFERENCES

1. Steenstra F, van Dijk CN. Achilles tendoscopy. Foot Ankle Clin N Am 2006;11: 429–38.
2. Kolodziej P, Glisson RR, Nunley JA. Risk of avulsion of the Achilles tendon after partial excision for treatment of insertional tendonitis and Haglund's deformity: a biomechanical study. Foot Ankle Int 1999;20(7):433–7.
3. Hamilton WB. Surgical anatomy of foot and ankle. Clin Symp 1985;37(3):2–32.
4. Komi PV. Relevance of in vivo force measurements to human biomechanics. J Biomech 1990;23(Suppl 1):23–34.
5. Sarrafian S. Functional anatomy of the foot and ankle. In: Sarrafian S, editor. Anatomy of the foot and ankle. Philadelphia: Lippincott-Raven; 1996. p. 255–72.
6. DiGiovanni CW, Kuo R, Tejwani N, et al. Isolated gastrocnemius tightness. J Bone Joint Surg Am 2002;84-A(6):962–70.
7. Whittle M. Gait analysis: an introduction. Oxford (United Kingdom): Butterworth-Heinemann; 1996.
8. Pinney SJ, Hansen ST, Sangeorzan BJ. The effect of ankle dorsiflexion on gastrocnemius recession. Foot Ankle Int 2002;23(1):26–9.
9. Lavery LA, Armstrong DG, Boulton AJ. Ankle equinus deformity and its relationship to high plantar pressure in a large population with diabetes mellitus. J Am Podiatr Med Assoc 2002;92(9):479–82.
10. Phisitkul P. Endoscopic surgery of the achilles tendon. Curr Rev Musculoskelet Med 2012;5:156–63.
11. Silfverskiöld N. Reduction of the uncrossed two-joint muscles of the leg to one-joint muscles in spastic conditions. Acta Chir Scand 1924;56:315–30.
12. Stotler WM, Van Bergeyk A, Manoli A. Preliminary results of gastrocnemius recession in adults. American Orthopaedic Foot and Ankle Society. Annual Summer meeting. Traverse City (MI), March 12, 2002.
13. Dietz FR, Albright JC, Dolan L. Medium term follow-up of the Achilles tendon lengthening in the treatment of ankle equinus in cerebral palsy. Iowa Orthop J 2006;26:27–32.
14. Mueller MJ, Sinacore DR, Hastings MK, et al. Effect of Achilles tendon lengthening on neuropathic plantar ulcers. A randomized clinical trial. J Bone Joint Surg Am 2003;85-A(8):1436–45.
15. Saxena A. Endoscopic gastrocnemius tenotomy. J Foot Ankle Surg 2002;41(1):57–8.
16. Eksin DW, Whiten S, Hillman SJ, et al. The conjoint junction of the triceps surae: implications for gastrocnemius tendon lengthening. Clin Anat 2007;20(8):924–8.
17. Tashjain RZ, Appel AL, Banerjee R, et al. Endoscopic gastrocnemius recession: evaluation in a cadaver model. Foot Ankle Int 2003;24(8):830–3.
18. Pinney SJ, Sangeorzan BJ, Hansen ST. Surgical anatomy of the gastrocnemius recession (Strayer procedure). Foot Ankle Int 2004;25(4):247–50.
19. Yeap EJ, Shamsul SA, Chong KW, et al. Simple two-portal technique for endoscopic gastrocnemius recession: clinical tip. Foot Ankle Int 2011;32(8):830–3.
20. Trevino S, Gibbs M, Panchbhavi V. Evaluation of results of endoscopic gastrocnemius recession. Foot Ankle Int 2005;26(5):359–64.
21. Angthong C, Kanitnate S. Dual-portal endoscopic gastrocnemius recession for the treatment of severe posttraumatic equinus deformity: a case series and review of technical modifications. J Nippon Med Sch 2012;79(3):198–203.
22. Carl T, Barrett SL. Cadaveric assessment of the gastrocnemius aponeurosis to assist in the pre-operative planning for two-portal endoscopic gastrocnemius recession. Foot 2005;15(3):137–40.

23. Tashjian RZ, Appel AJ, Banerjee R, et al. Anatomic study of the gastrocnemius-soleus junction and it relationship to the sural nerve. Foot Ankle Int 2003;24(6):473–6.
24. Grady JF, Kelly C. Endoscopic gastrocnemius recession for treating equinus in pediatric patients. Clin Orthop Relat Res 2010;468:1033–8.
25. Roukis MH, Schweinberger MH. Complications associated with uni-portal endoscopic gastrocnemius recession in a diabetic patient population: an observational case series. J Foot Ankle Surg 2010;49:68–70.
26. Saxena A, Widtfeldt A. Endoscopic gastrocnemius recession: preliminary report on 18 cases. J Foot Ankle Surg 2004;43(5):302–6.
27. Saxena A, Widfeldt A. Endoscopic gastrocnemius ressesion as therapy for gastrocnemius equinus. Z Orthop Unfall 2007;145(4):499–504 [in German].
28. Leppilahti J, Puranan J, Orava S. Incidence of Achilles tendon rupture. Acta Orthop Scand 1996;67:277–9.
29. Suchak A, Bostick G, Reid S, et al. The incidence of Achilles ruptures in Edmonton, Canada. Foot Ankle Int 2005;26:932–6.
30. Wong J, Barrass V, Maffulli N. Quantitative review of operative and nonoperative management of Achilles tendon ruptures. Am J Sports Med 2002;30:565–75.
31. Khan RJ, Fick D, Keogh A, et al. Treatment of acute Achilles tendon ruptures. A metanalysis of randomized, controlled trials. J Bone Joint Surg Am 2005;87:2202–10.
32. Moller M, Movin T, Granhed H, et al. Acute rupture of tendo Achilles: a prospective, randomized study of comparison between surgical and non-surgical treatment. J Bone Joint Surg 2001;83:843–8.
33. Ma GW, Griffith TG. Percutaneous repair of acute closed ruptured Achilles tendon: a new technique. Clin Orthop Relat Res 1977;(128):247–55.
34. Fortis AP, Dimas A, Lamprakis A. Repair of Achilles tendon rupture under endoscopic control. Arthroscopy 2008;24(6):683–8.
35. Turgut A, Gunal I, Maralcan G, et al. Endoscopy, assisted percutaneous repair of the Achilles tendon ruptures: a cadaveric and clinical study. Knee Surg Sports Traumatol Arthrosc 2002;10(2):130–3.
36. Halasi T, Tallay A, Berkes I. Percutaneous Achilles tendon repair with and without endoscopic control. Knee Surg Sports Traumatol Arthrosc 2003;11(6):409–14.
37. Tang KI, Thermann H, Dai G, et al. Arthroscopically assisted percutaneous repair of fresh closed achilles tendon rupture by Kessler's suture. Am J Sports Med 2007;35(4):589–96.
38. Doral MN, Bozkurt M, Turhan E, et al. Percutaneous suturing of the ruptured Achilles tendon with endoscopic control. Arch Orthop Trauma Surg 2009;129(8):1093–101.
39. Gossage W, Kohls-Gatzoulis J, Solan M. Endoscopic assisted repair of chronic Achilles tendon rupture with flexor hallucis longus augmentation. Foot Ankle Int 2010;31(4):344–7.
40. Lui TH. Endoscopic assisted flexor hallucis tendon transfer in the management of chronic rupture of Achilles tendon. Knee Surg Sports Traumatol Arthrosc 2007;15:1163–6.
41. Haglund P. Beitrag zur Klinik der Achillessehne. Z Orthop Chir 1928;49:49–58.
42. Sammarco GJ, Taylor L. Operative management of Haglund's deformity in the nonathlete: a retrospective study. Foot Ankle Int 1998;19:724–9.
43. Labib SA, Pendleton AM. Endoscopic calcaneoplasty: an improved technique. J Surg Orthop Adv 2012;21(3):176–80.
44. Ortmann FW, McBryde AM. Endoscopic bony and soft-tissue decompression of the retrocalcaneal space for the treatment of Haglund's deformity and retrocalcaneal bursitis. Foot Ankle Int 2007;28(2):149–53.

45. van Dijk CN, van Dyk CE, Scholten PE, et al. Endoscopic calcaneoplasty. Am J Sports Med 2001;29:185–9.
46. van Sterkenburg MN, Muller B, Mass M, et al. Apperance of the weight-bearing lateral radiograph in retrocalcaneal bursitits. Acta Orthop 2010;81(3):387–90.
47. Jerosch J, Schunk J, Sokkar SH. Endoscopic calcaneoplasty (ECP) as a surgical treatment of Haglund's syndrome. Knee Surg Sports Traumatol Arthrosc 2007;15: 927–34.
48. Lysholm J, Wiklander J. Injuries in runners. Am J Sports Med 1987;15(2):168–71.
49. Segesser B, Goesele A, Rengli P. The Achilles tendon in sports. Orthopade 1995; 24(3):252–67.
50. Maffulli N, Binfield PM, Moore D, et al. Surgical decompression of chronic central core lesions of the Achilles tendon. Am J Sports Med 1999;27(6):747–52.
51. Lui TH. Treatment of chronic noninsertional Achilles tendinopathy with endoscopic Achilles tendon debridement and flexor hallucis longus transfer. Foot Ankle Spec 2012;5(3):195–200.
52. Maquirriain J. Surgical treatment of chronic Achilles tendinopathy: long-term results of the endoscopic technique. J Foot Ankle Surg 2013;52:451–5.

Anterior Ankle Arthroscopy
Indications, Pitfalls, and Complications

David M. Epstein, MD[a,b,*], Brandee S. Black, MD, MEd[c],
Seth L. Sherman, MD[c]

KEYWORDS

- Ankle arthroscopy • Anterior ankle arthroscopy • Indications • Complications
- Pitfalls • Technique

KEY POINTS

- Anterior ankle arthroscopy is a comprehensive tool for diagnosis and treatment of a diverse range of ankle pathologies.
- Indications are expanding with improved surgical technique and instrumentation and include management of instability, impingement, osteochondritis dissecans lesions, chondral lesions, fractures, synovitis and loose bodies.
- Knowledge of ankle anatomy and biomechanics is critical to avoid iatrogenic complications.
- The complication rate of anterior ankle arthroscopy ranges from 3.4% to 9%; most common complications include neurologic injury to the superficial peroneal nerve and superficial infection.

INDICATIONS

Anterior ankle arthroscopy is indicated for the diagnosis and treatment of a broad spectrum of common ankle disorders (**Box 1**).[1] Over the past few decades, advances in operative techniques and arthroscopic instrumentation have allowed these

Dr S.L. Sherman is a Committee Member for the American Orthopedic Society for Sports Medicine and the Arthroscopy Association of North America; he is a Consultant for Regeneration Technologies, Inc, and Arthrex, Inc (unpaid); he has grant support from Arthrex, Inc; and is an editorial/governing board member for the American Journal of Orthopedics and Arthroscopy. Dr D.M. Epstein is a Consultant for Stryker Orthopedics. Dr B.S. Black has no disclosures. No commercial company has any direct financial interest in the subject matter or materials discussed in this article.
 a Tri-County Orthopedics & Sports Medicine, 197 Ridgedale Avenue, Suite 300, Cedar Knolls, NJ 07927, USA; b Morristown Medical Center, 100, Madison Avenue, Morristown, NJ 07960, USA; c Department of Orthopaedic Surgery, University of Missouri, 1100 Virginia Avenue, Columbia, MO 65212, USA
* Corresponding author.
E-mail address: drdeps@gmail.com

Foot Ankle Clin N Am 20 (2015) 41–57
http://dx.doi.org/10.1016/j.fcl.2014.10.001
1083-7515/15/$ – see front matter © 2015 Elsevier Inc. All rights reserved.

> **Box 1**
> **Indications in foot and ankle arthroscopy**
>
> Ankle impingement
>   Bony impingement
>   Soft tissue impingement
> Osteochondral lesions
> Ankle instability
> Removal of loose bodies
> Assessing fracture reduction
>   Evaluating for chondral injury
>   Evaluating for syndesmosis injury
> Arthrofibrosis
> Arthritis
> Chronic synovitis

indications to expand to include rare or complex injury patterns. Ankle arthroscopy—compared with open procedures in the foot and ankle—allows for preservation of the soft tissue envelope, thus accelerating a return to daily activities and athletic endeavors.[2–5] Additionally, diagnostic arthroscopy has proven to be a valuable tool in the comprehensive treatment of many foot and ankle injuries.[1,6–10] A recent study by Amendola and Bonasia[11] revealed arthroscopy to be more sensitive when compared with preoperative physical examination and imaging in diagnosing chondral injury in the chronically unstable ankle (50% vs 4% sensitivity).

A systematic review by Glazebrook and colleagues[12] found fair, evidence-based literature to support a recommendation for the use of ankle arthroscopy for the treatment of ankle impingement and osteochondral lesions and also as an adjunct to ankle arthrodesis. Although commonly used, less support is found in the literature for routine use of arthroscopy for ankle instability, septic arthritis, arthrofibrosis, and removal of loose bodies. The authors concluded that insufficient evidence exists to support or refute the benefit of arthroscopy for the management of ankle fractures.

The use of ankle arthroscopy for the management of ankle and talus fractures can be valuable at the time of reduction and fixation (**Fig. 1**). Advantages of arthroscopically assisted internal fixation for talus fractures include improved anatomic exposure with the potential for reduced postoperative infection and skin necrosis, better visualization of the articular surface for fracture reduction, and preservation of blood supply. Potential disadvantages include increased surgical time, soft tissue swelling, and challenging surgical technique.[13,14]

Arthroscopically assisted internal reduction for ankle fractures—as well as evaluation of chondral damage after ankle fracture fixation—have been described with minimal adverse sequelae. Arthroscopic evaluation of 9 ankle joints after either supination–external rotation or pronation–external rotation fractures identified 8 patients with articular cartilage damage to the talar dome that was not identified on preoperative imaging.[15] Additionally, a retrospective review from Leontaritis and colleagues[16] found that, among 84 patients treated with open reduction internal fixation along with ankle arthroscopy, 61 (73%) had intra-articular chondral lesions.

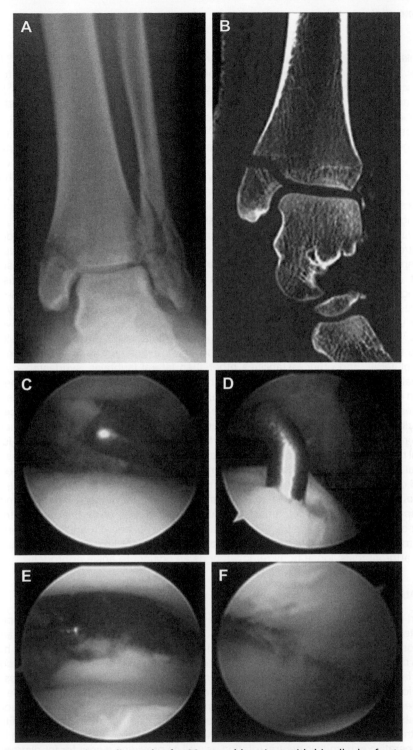

Fig. 1. Anteroposterior radiograph of a 20-year-old patient with bimalleolar fracture (*A*). Compute tomography shows loose fragments in tibiotalar joint (*B*). Intraoperative photos show removal of loose body (*C*), osteochondral lesion of the lateral talus (*D*), and assessment of preoperative (*E*) and postoperative (*F*) reduction.

Ankle arthroscopy can also aid the diagnosis of syndesmotic injury (**Fig. 2**).[16] In a study by Ono and colleagues,[17] the use of arthroscopic diagnosis was found to be as accurate as the squeeze test in diagnosing diastasis of the distal tibiofibular joint after ankle fracture. The authors detected instability of the joint by a squeeze test under fluoroscopy or by residual, arthroscopically appreciated diastasis of the joint. In a prospective study by Lui and colleagues,[18] 53 ankle fractures without preoperative radiographic evidence of syndesmosis diastasis were assessed with intraoperative stress radiography and arthroscopy. The tibiofibular syndesmosis was found to be unstable by intraoperative stress radiography in 30.2% of the patients and, by arthroscopy, 66% of patients were found to have instability. The authors concluded that ankle arthroscopy was superior to intraoperative stress radiography in detecting syndesmosis disruption in their patient population.

Treatment for lateral ankle instability most commonly consists of the open modified Brostrom procedure after routine arthroscopic joint inspection. Ankle arthroscopy is an important component that allows for confirmation of an instability pattern, assessment of the anterior talofibular ligament tissue quality, treatment of soft tissue impingement, syndesmosis injury, and concomitant osteochondral lesions.[6] Before lateral ligament reconstruction, evaluation of the joint first by ankle arthroscopy has been useful to find secondary pathology that may be contributing to ankle symptoms.[19] Associated pathology can include intra-articular pathology (chondral lesions, loose bodies, ossicles, synovitis, and arthrosis), impingement lesions (anterior and anterolateral), and other instabilities other than lateral (subtalar, syndesmotic, and medial).[11] Hinterman and colleagues[20] found that intra-articular pathology, a chondral lesion of the talus specifically, was found arthroscopically in more than 50% of cases, whereas the preoperative diagnosis was made in only 4% of patients. Recently described "all-inside" arthroscopic techniques of lateral ankle ligament reconstruction have reported good results. Cottom and Rigby[21] reveal excellent clinical and functional results after 1 year of follow-up in treating a cohort of 40 patients with "all-inside" lateral ligament reconstructions with suture anchors. Others have similarly reported good outcomes after long-term follow-up using a similar technique.[22,23]

In our practice, indications for anterior ankle arthroscopy include diagnostic and/or therapeutic arthroscopy before lateral ankle ligament repair or reconstruction, treatment of chondral lesions in the setting of ankle fractures, anterior ankle impingement syndrome, osteochondritis dissecans lesions of the talus or tibia, inflammatory synovitis, arthrofibrosis, loose body removal, or as an adjunct to ankle arthrodesis.

PITFALLS

When performing anterior ankle arthroscopy, careful planning and meticulous operative technique helps to prevent potential pitfalls (**Box 2**). Although anterior ankle arthroscopy is most commonly performed in the supine position, techniques have been described with the use of the lateral decubitus and prone positions for concomitant lateral or posterior arthroscopy. Supine positioning allows for easy access for anterior ankle arthroscopy and the placement of posterior ankle portals if needed. A padded thigh support allows for positioning of the ankle about 2 fingerbreadths above the table (**Fig. 3**). A noninvasive distractor is placed about the ankle (**Fig. 4**). Additionally, the judicious use of a beanbag underneath the posterior thigh can serve to hold the operative extremity in neutral rotation as well as providing a counter for distraction across the ankle joint (**Fig. 5**). During positioning for surgery, care must be taken to position the patient as proximal on the operating room table as possible to allow for adequate room for ankle distraction with the external traction device. An improperly

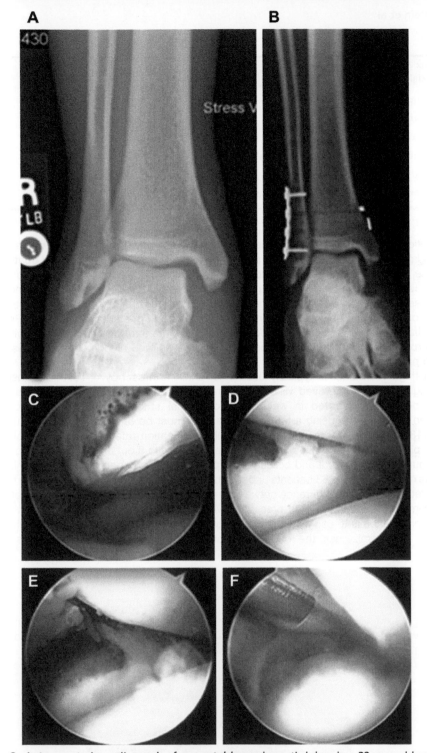

Fig. 2. Anteroposterior radiograph of an unstable syndesmotic injury in a 22-year-old collegiate soccer player before (*A*) and after syndesmotic fixation (*B*). Arthroscopic pictures demonstrate synovitis and hemorrhage within the joint (*C*) and syndesmosis (*D*) with instability to intraoperative stress (*E*) confirmed with probing (*F*).

Box 2
Pitfalls in foot and ankle arthroscopy

Setup

Tourniquet

Traction and/or ankle position

Identifying surface anatomy for portal placement

Fluid management during arthroscopy

Arthroscopic reach in using the standard anterior ankle portals

---

positioned patient can compromise the effectiveness of the manual ankle distractor. The lateral decubitus position can afford access to the anterior, lateral, and posterior ankle.[19] A beanbag is used for stability, an axillary role is placed, and all bony prominences are well padded. The hip is abducted, the knee is flexed, and then the knee is placed in an arthroscopic knee holder to support the thigh for the anterior ankle arthroscopy. The knee holder is removed for lateral and posterior arthroscopy. Prone positioning allows access to the posterior ankle joints and the anterior ankle joint.[24] Gel roles are placed to support the chest and pelvis, and all bony prominences are well padded.

A thigh tourniquet is typically used with ankle arthroscopy.[25] Tourniquet use is thought to allow improved visibility and reduce operative time. However, this has not been demonstrated in well-designed clinical studies on ankle arthroscopy. When applying and using a tourniquet, caution must be taken. In a national survey of 118,590 knee arthroscopies, the overall complication rate was 0.8%. Neurologic complications compromised 6.8% of these insults, with 8 out of 10 directly attributed to tourniquet use. Zaidi and colleagues[26] performed a prospective, nonrandomized, case control study on 63 patients undergoing ankle arthroscopy with or without a tourniquet, and found no difference between groups with respect to duration of operation, maximum intraoperative fluid pressures, visibility, and postoperative complications. Our preference is to use a well-placed thigh tourniquet during anterior ankle arthroscopy. To minimize risk, the tourniquet should be elevated for the minimum possible

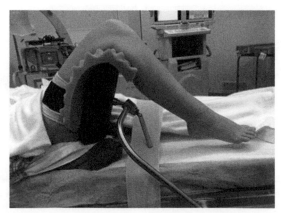

Fig. 3. Supine positioning for anterior ankle arthroscopy using an arthroscopic knee well-leg holder.

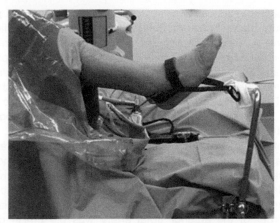

Fig. 4. Supine positioning with an arthroscopic knee well-leg holder in place and a noninvasive ankle distracter.

duration (<2 hours) and lowest pressure (ie, 250 mm Hg) to maintain adequate hemostasis.

Different methods to facilitate visualization during ankle arthroscopy have been described. Methods to create joint distraction include the use of ankle straps, a calcaneal pin, invasive distracters, and a fracture table.[27] Invasive distractors carry risks of pin-track infections, fracture of the fibula, stress fracture of the tibia, pin breakage, ligament damage, and neurovascular injury.[28] Rarely are invasive distractors used for ankle arthroscopy, because noninvasive methods allow for adequate distraction.[29]

Two noninvasive methods—distraction of the ankle with a strap or the dorsiflexion method—have been evaluated clinically. Lozano-Calderon and colleagues[30] prospectively evaluated the ease of visualization of anatomic structures according to Ferkel's 21-point ankle arthroscopy protocol with and without traction. In his study of 103 patients, he evaluated arthroscopically the joint without traction using the dorsiflexion method and gave one point for each area that was well visualized up to a maximum of 21 points. He then repeated arthroscopy with a noninvasive distractor in place and repeated the scoring. A significant difference in the ease of visualization using

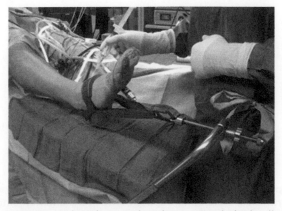

Fig. 5. Supine positioning. A beanbag under the proximal thigh allows for resistance against the noninvasive ankle distracter and neutral rotation of the operative extremity.

noninvasive distraction, especially for structures in the central and posterior ankle, was found. Although noninvasive traction was better overall, dorsiflexion improved visualization of the anterior compartment and lateral gutters. Zengerink and van Dijk[28] reviewed retrospectively complications of 1305 consecutive patients who underwent anterior and/or posterior ankle arthroscopy by the dorsiflexion method. The overall complication rate was 3.5%. The complication rate for hindfoot endoscopy alone was 2.3%. The most common complication, namely, neurologic injury, occurred at a rate of 1.9%, which compares favorably with the 5.4% neurologic complication rate in another study that used continuous distraction.[31]

In a cadaveric study by de Leeuw and colleagues,[32] 6 fresh frozen ankle specimens amputated above the knee were analyzed to determine the distance between the anterior distal tibial and the overlying anterior neurovascular structures. A significant difference in distance was found when dorsiflexion versus distraction was used. The median distance between the anterior border of the inferior tibial articular facet and posterior border of the anterior tibial artery was 0.9 cm in dorsiflexion and 0.7 cm in distraction (**Fig. 6**). Therefore, the authors concluded that the distracted ankle position risks iatrogenic damage to the neurovascular structures when performing anterior ankle arthroscopy.

When used safely, noninvasive ankle distraction, can allow for an increased field of view.[32] To determine safe distraction forces and length of time that traction was applied, Dowdy and colleagues[33] studied 14 ankles without foot and ankle pathology. The study included healthy volunteers where in-line traction was applied to the ankle at varying forces and lengths of time. Sensory nerve amplitudes as well as subjective paresthesias were recorded. The authors recommend that up to 135 N (30 lb) of traction can be applied for up to 1 hour. Greater forces and distraction maintained for more than 1 hour are associated with irreversible nerve conduction changes.

Arthroscopes for the ankle joint vary in size, ranging from 1.9 to 4.0 mm in diameter. A 30° arthroscope typically allows adequate visualization of the anterior ankle joint, although a 70° arthroscope may allow for improved visualization in a tight joint space. Separate inflow and outflow portals allow optimal joint distension. Pump or gravity

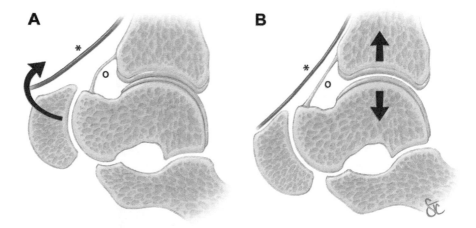

Fig. 6. Relationship between the anterior joint capsule, O, and the neurovascular structures. With the ankle dorsiflexed, there is more space between the anterior joint capsule and the anterior neurovascular structures. (*A*) With the ankle in a noninvasive distraction device, the space is narrower (*B*). The anterior neurovascular structures (*asterix*).

systems for fluid management may be used, but pump systems increase the risk of fluid extravasation into the surrounding soft tissues. This can lead to increased compartment pressures and ischemia. Hanson and Varner[34] describe a technique for decreasing fluid extravasation during arthroscopy of the ankle. After the portal locations are marked on the skin, a 4-inch Coban dressing is snuggly wrapped in 2 layers from the midfoot to the distal leg. The forefoot is wrapped separately to ensure maintenance of sterile technique. The portal sites are located and small openings are created through the Coban. The authors have found that this technique limits soft tissue edema after ankle arthroscopy. We find that the use of a 2.7-mm, 30° arthroscope permits safe access into and maneuverability within the joint with minimal risk of iatrogenic injury.

The primary working portals for anterior ankle arthroscopy are the anteromedial (medial to the tibialis anterior tendon) and anterolateral (lateral to the peroneus tertius, or if not present, lateral to the extensor digitorum longus tendon) portals. Marking the surface anatomy can be helpful in identifying and avoiding the neurovascular structures at risk (**Fig. 7**). The greater saphenous vein and saphenous

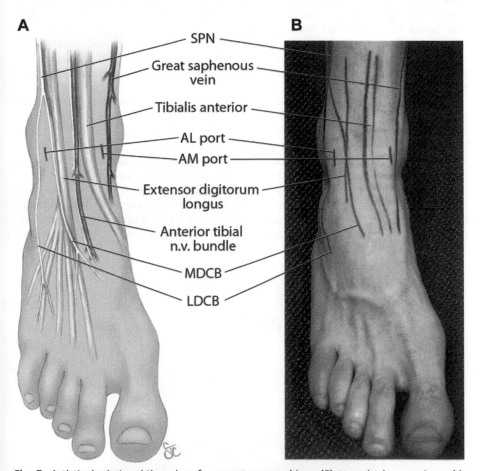

Fig. 7. Artist's depiction (A) and surface anatomy markings (B) to assist in anterior ankle arthroscopy portal placement. AL port, anterolateral portal; AM port, anteromedial portal; LDCB, lateral dorsal cutaneous branch of the SPN; MDCB, medial dorsal cutaneous branch of the SPN; n.v., neurovascular; SPN, superficial peroneal nerve.

nerve can be injured while establishing the anteromedial portal. An anatomic study of 16 cadaveric ankles mapped the courses of the saphenous nerve and greater saphenous vein.[35] The authors determined that the anteromedial portal should be more than 1 cm from the anterior aspect of the medial malleolus to avoid injury to the greater saphenous vein. The superficial peroneal nerve (SPN) and its branches are at risk with anterolateral portal placement. Cadaver studies have shown that 33% of specimens can have accessory branches of the SPN, which may predispose this nerve to iatrogenic injury.[36] Another consideration is that the SPN is most easily visualized, and thus marked, with the ankle in plantar flexion and inversion (**Fig. 8**). Once the ankle is dorsiflexed with neutral version, and then placed in a noninvasive distraction strap, the course of the nerve has been shown to move laterally.[37] Therefore, safe anterolateral portal placement is just medial to the marking of the SPN course. Anatomic variation or improper positioning of the anterolateral portal has been suggested to be responsible for injury to the anterior tibial artery, including pseudoaneurysm.[38–40] In our practice, needle localization and initial saline joint insufflation assist with portal placement and increase safe distance from the overlying neurovascular structures. The anteromedial portal is established first, because this portal has a decreased risk of neurovascular injury. The anterolateral portal is then established with an outside-in technique under direct arthroscopic visualization. The skin and subcutaneous tissue are incised and blunt dissection is utilized to minimize risk of iatrogenic nerve injury.

There is substantial risk of iatrogenic cartilage damage upon introducing arthroscopic instruments into the joint.[29] Small-gauge needles and blunt trocars should be used to establish the portals. Proper portal placement with a trajectory parallel to the tibial plafond can reduce iatrogenic injury to the articular cartilage. The use of intraoperative mini–C-arm fluoroscopy has been suggested to ensure that the appropriate angle is used while applying the least amount of distraction necessary.[41]

Arthroscopically assisted treatment of talar dome cartilage defects has been described.[42–44] The appropriateness of arthroscopy in reaching talar osteochondral lesions can be estimated based on geographic location of the lesion on computed tomography. The anterior defect border is the landmark for accessibility because only

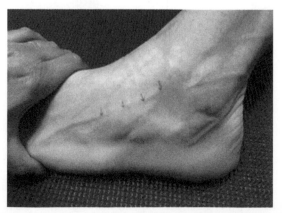

Fig. 8. Plantar flexion and inversion of the ankle to visualize the intermediate dorsal cutaneous branch of the superficial peroneal nerve. The anterolateral portal should be placed medial to the marking of this structure.

this part of the defect has to be identified initially during arthroscopy. This was shown by van Bergen and colleagues[45] in a study of 59 ankles. Preoperative computed tomography was obtained and custom software calculated the percentage of the talus visible through standard arthroscopic portals. Almost one half of the talar dome is accessible anterior to the anterior distal tibial rim, 48.2% of the medial talar dome and 47.8% of the lateral talar dome. However, the authors point out that, with greater plantar flexion, the area visible is greater, and this was an important independent predictive factor in arthroscopic reach. The "arthroscopic reach" of nearly 50% of the anterior talar dome limits treatment of talar defects extending far into the posterior talar dome. These lesions can be addressed with a combined posterolateral portal or a 2-portal hindfoot arthroscopic approach.[46,47]

Preoperative evaluation with MRI or computed tomography can be valuable in determining the accessibility of an osteochondral lesion with an arthroscopic approach. Surgical planning may include the possibility of conversion to an open anterior approach, or may mandate the use of a malleolar osteotomy for adequate exposure. The patient should be counseled effectively regarding these preoperative considerations.

COMPLICATIONS

Overall, the average complication rate in anterior ankle arthroscopy has been reported to be between 3.4% and 9%.[47,48] Complications such as neurologic, tendon, and ligament injuries, wound complications, infection, and instrument breakage can occur in foot and ankle arthroscopy (**Box 3**). The most common complication is

---

Box 3
Complications in foot and ankle arthroscopy

Nerve injury

    Superficial peroneal nerve and its branches

    Deep peroneal nerve

    Sural and saphenous nerves

Vascular injury

    Pseudoaneurysm of the anterior tibial artery

    Pseudoaneurysm of the dorsalis pedis artery

Infection

Hemarthrosis

Deep vein thrombosis

Synovial fistula

Tendon Injury

    Rupture of the extensor halluces longes

    Rupture of the extensor digitorum communis

Failure of procedure

    Recurrent instability

    Nonunion or malunion after fracture fixation

Persistent pain

neurologic injury, with the SPN being the most commonly injured nerve.[48] The dorsiflexion method for anterior ankle arthroscopy has been evaluated and suggested to decrease the overall complication rate to 3.5%, with the incidence of neurologic injury at 1.9%.[28] In a recent systematic review, the overall complication rate in ankle arthroscopy for anterolateral impingement using the standard 2-portal technique was 4%.[49]

The SPN is the most at-risk structure in anterior ankle arthroscopy. Inadvertent placement of the anterolateral portal risks iatrogenic injury to the nerve or one of its branches. Anatomic studies at the talocrural joint have shown that the majority of people, 52.9%, have 2 branches of the SPN, namely, the intermediate dorsal cutaneous nerve (also known as Lemont's nerve), and the medial dorsal cutaneous nerve.[50] Another anatomic study found that the number of SPN branches crossing the ankle joint varied from 1 to 5 per specimen and the width of the branches varied from 1 and 13 mm.[51] Identifying and marking the SPN and its branches preoperatively has been shown to be an effective method in decrease iatrogenic injury. In a study of 96 consecutively treated patients with mean follow-up of 25.3 months, 1.04% of the patients were found to have sensory loss localized to the distribution of the medial dorsal cutaneous branch of the SPN after ankle arthroscopy with preoperative marking of the SPN and its branches.[52]

The deep peroneal, sural, and saphenous nerves are less commonly injured during anterior ankle arthroscopy. In a case series of 260 patients, Deng and colleagues[39] reported the incidence of deep peroneal, sural, and saphenous nerve injury to be 0.77%, 0.38%, and 0.38%, respectively. In establishing the anteromedial portal, others have described a less than 1% incidence of injury to the saphenous nerve.[53]

Vascular injury is possible during anterior ankle arthroscopy. There are many reports of pseudoaneurysm of the anterior tibial artery, and 1 report of pseudoaneurysm of the dorsalis pedis artery after anterior ankle arthroscopy in the literature.[38,40,54–58] In cadaveric studies, a 4.3% rate of anatomic variation of the anterior tibial artery and dorsalis pedis artery was shown.[59] A study by Son and colleagues[38] used MRI to better estimate the rate of anatomic variation near the anterolateral portal. The authors found that the 2 most at-risk variations of the anterior tibial artery and its branches were a location lateral to the extensor digitorum longus and posterior tibialis tendons or in the typical region of safety for the anterolateral ankle portal. These 2 anatomic variants occurred in 22 of 358 cases (6.2%).

Infection is a potential complication in any operative procedure. The incidence of infection after knee arthroscopy, the most commonly performed procedure by orthopedic surgeons, is 0.84%.[60] Ferkel and colleagues[48] reported 8 superficial infections in 612 ankle arthroscopies (0.13%). Those infections were attributed to the absence of a cannula for instrumentation, the use of Steri-strips too close the wound and early mobilization of the joint after surgery.[29]

Postoperative hemarthrosis is a possible complication after anterior ankle arthroscopy. The frequency of this adverse event is rarely reported, but in 1 study it was found to be the third most common minor complication, occurring at a rate of 0.3%.[49] These authors considered hemarthrosis a minor complication, because all cases resolved without adverse long-term effects at least 12 months postoperatively. Deflating the tourniquet to ensure adequate hemostasis may help to avoid such a complication.

Venous thromboembolism (VTE) has been reported after arthroscopic surgery of the shoulder and knee, but limited studies report the incidence after hip or ankle arthroscopy.[61] In a systematic review of 8 publications, the incidence of VTE after foot and ankle injury treated conservatively and surgically has been reported to be 5.9% and 3.3%, respectively.[62] However, among the 2 groups, 85.6% of the conservatively treated group and 92.9% of the surgically treated group were asymptomatic. The normal postoperative course can mimic the symptoms of VTE, unilateral swelling, and calf pain, which make diagnosing a VTE even more challenging. Identifying high-risk individuals before ankle arthroscopy can guide the surgeon in the decision to provide VTE prophylaxis in the postoperative period. We do not currently recommend VTE chemoprophylaxis for patients after anterior ankle arthroscopy unless the patient has a substantially elevated preoperative thrombotic risk.

Sinus tract formation can occur in chronically draining ankle arthroscopy portals. In 1305 ankle arthroscopies, Zengerink and van Dijk[28] reported 7 patients to have developed synovial fistulas at the portal sites. In a consecutive series of 105 patients by Rasmussen and Jensen,[63] 1 synovial fistula developed, which responded to arthroscopic synovectomy and intravenous antibiotics. The authors do not speculate on why fistulas developed, but careful closure of the portals with prompt treatment of persistent drainage can assist with the prevention of synovial tract formation. Application of a well-padded postoperative splint and decreased early ankle mobilization until wound healing may help to decrease the incidence of this complication.

Rupture of the extensor halluces longus and extensor digitorum communis tendons have been reported in the postoperative period after anterior ankle arthroscopy.[64,65] The use of radiofrequency ablation and aggressive debridement with a shaver in the anterior ankle joint has been attributed to causing iatrogenic delayed rupture of the extensor tendons. Injury to the anterior talofibular ligament or the deltoid can occur when placing accessory anterolateral or anteromedial portals.[29] Careful portal placement and judicious work under direct visualization in the anterior ankle joint can assist in avoiding these complications.

Less commonly reported complications in anterior ankle arthroscopy are complex regional pain syndrome, instrument breakage, and iatrogenic excision of the distal fibula.[28,29,66] Complex regional pain syndrome can develop after any trauma and/or operative procedure. Symptoms include spontaneous pain out of proportion to a stimulus, edema, calor, and sweating in the ankle region. Appropriately sized baskets and graspers designed to break at the handle and not at the tip should be used to prevent escape of the broken piece within the joint. Last, a thorough understanding of the intra-articular and extra-articular anatomy of the ankle joint will aid in preventing iatrogenic injury to nearby anatomic structures.

Failure of the procedure, including recurrent instability, nonunion or malunion, and persistent pain, are risks with anterior ankle arthroscopy. Prognostic factors contributing to a poor outcome include chondral lesions, advanced age, and history of a previous trauma.[67] Careful surgical indications based on thorough history, physical examination, and appropriate imaging studies will help to minimize the risk of surgical failure.

SUMMARY

Anterior ankle arthroscopy is a minimally invasive operative procedure that can be useful for a variety of ankle conditions. With careful preoperative planning and meticulous operative technique, common pitfalls and complications can be avoided. As instrumentation improves and surgical experience broadens, it is likely that ankle arthroscopy will be utilized for a growing number of pathologic conditions. Few controlled, prospective studies have evaluated the efficacy of anterior ankle arthroscopy for common and complex ankle condition. Future research is warranted to validate these arthroscopic techniques and to increase the safety margin for our patients.

REFERENCES

1. Hepple S, Guha A. The role of ankle arthroscopy in acute ankle injuries of the athlete. Foot Ankle Clin 2013;18:185–94.
2. Abdelatif NM. Combined arthroscopic management of concurrent posterior and anterior ankle pathologies. Knee Surg Sports Traumatol Arthrosc 2014;22:2837–42.
3. van Eekeren IC, Reilingh ML, van Dijk CN. Rehabilitation and return-to-sports activity after debridement and bone marrow stimulation of osteochondral talar defects. Sports Med 2012;42:857–70.
4. van Bergen CJ, Kox LS, Maas M, et al. Arthroscopic treatment of osteochondral defects of the talus: outcomes at eight to twenty years of follow-up. J Bone Joint Surg Am 2013;95:519–25.
5. Phisitkul P, Tennant JN, Amendola A. Is there any value to arthroscopic debridement of ankle osteoarthritis and impingement? Foot Ankle Clin 2013;18:449–58.
6. Guillo S, Bauer T, Lee JW, et al. Consensus in chronic ankle instability: aetiology, assessment, surgical indications and place for arthroscopy. Orthop Traumatol Surg Res 2013;99:S411–9.
7. Cychosz CC, Phisitkul P, Barg A, et al. Foot and ankle tendoscopy: evidence-based recommendations. Arthroscopy 2014;30:755–65.
8. Bare A, Ferkel RD. Peroneal tendon tears: associated arthroscopic findings and results after repair. Arthroscopy 2009;25:1288–97.
9. Kerr HL, Bayley E, Jackson R, et al. The role of arthroscopy in the treatment of functional instability of the ankle. Foot Ankle Surg 2013;19:273–5.
10. Lui TH. Arthroscopy and endoscopy of the foot and ankle: indications for new techniques. Arthroscopy 2007;23:889–902.
11. Amendola A, Bonasia DE. When is ankle arthroscopy indicated in ankle instability? Oper Tech Sports Med 2010;18:2–10.
12. Glazebrook MA, Ganapathy V, Bridge MA, et al. Evidence-based indications for ankle arthroscopy. Arthroscopy 2009;25:1478–90.
13. Hsu AR, Gross CE, Lee S, et al. Extended indications for foot and ankle arthroscopy. J Am Acad Orthop Surg 2014;22:10–9.
14. Bonasia DE, Rossi R, Saltzman CL, et al. The role of arthroscopy in the management of fractures about the ankle. J Am Acad Orthop Surg 2011;19:226–35.
15. Thordarson DB, Bains R, Shepherd LE. The role of ankle arthroscopy on the surgical management of ankle fractures. Foot Ankle Int 2001;22:123–5.
16. Leontaritis N, Hinojosa L, Panchbhavi VK. Arthroscopically detected intra-articular lesions associated with acute ankle fractures. J Bone Joint Surg Am 2009;91:333–9.
17. Ono A, Nishikawa S, Nagao A, et al. Arthroscopically assisted treatment of ankle fractures: arthroscopic findings and surgical outcomes. Arthroscopy 2004;20:627–31.
18. Lui TH, Ip K, Chow HT. Comparison of radiologic and arthroscopic diagnoses of distal tibiofibular syndesmosis disruption in acute ankle fracture. Arthroscopy 2005;21:1370.
19. Hampton CB, Shawen SB, Keeling JJ. Positioning technique for combined anterior, lateral, and posterior ankle and hindfoot procedures: technique tip. Foot Ankle Int 2010;31:348–50.

20. Hintermann B, Boss A, Schafer D. Arthroscopic findings in patients with chronic ankle instability. Am J Sports Med 2002;30:402–9.
21. Cottom JM, Rigby RB. The "all inside" arthroscopic Brostrom procedure: a prospective study of 40 consecutive patients. J Foot Ankle Surg 2013;52:568–74.
22. Corte-Real NM, Moreira RM. Arthroscopic repair of chronic lateral ankle instability. Foot Ankle Int 2009;30:213–7.
23. Nery C, Raduan F, Del Buono A, et al. Arthroscopic-assisted Brostrom-Gould for chronic ankle instability: a long-term follow-up. Am J Sports Med 2011;39:2381–8.
24. Kim HN, Park YJ, Lee SY, et al. Three-portal ankle arthroscopy in prone position with ankle suspended: technique tip. Foot Ankle Int 2012;33:1027–30.
25. Zhang Y, Li L, Wang J, et al. Do patients benefit from tourniquet in arthroscopic surgeries of the knee? Knee Surg Sports Traumatol Arthrosc 2013;21:1125–30.
26. Zaidi R, Hasan K, Sharma A, et al. Ankle arthroscopy: a study of tourniquet versus no tourniquet. Foot Ankle Int 2014;35:478–82.
27. Waseem M, Barrie JL. A new distraction method in difficult ankle arthroscopy. J Foot Ankle Surg 2002;41:412–3.
28. Zengerink M, van Dijk CN. Complications in ankle arthroscopy. Knee Surg Sports Traumatol Arthrosc 2012;20:1420–31.
29. Carlson MJ, Ferkel RD. Complications in ankle and foot arthroscopy. Sports Med Arthrosc 2013;21:135–9.
30. Lozano-Calderon SA, Samocha Y, McWilliam J. Comparative performance of ankle arthroscopy with and without traction. Foot Ankle Int 2012;33:740–5.
31. Young BH, Flanigan RM, DiGiovanni BF. Complications of ankle arthroscopy utilizing a contemporary noninvasive distraction technique. J Bone Joint Surg Am 2011;93:963–8.
32. de Leeuw PA, Golanó P, Clavero JA, et al. Anterior ankle arthroscopy, distraction or dorsiflexion? Knee Surg Sports Traumatol Arthrosc 2010;18:594–600.
33. Dowdy PA, Watson BV, Amendola A, et al. Noninvasive ankle distraction: relationship between force, magnitude of distraction, and nerve conduction abnormalities. Arthroscopy 1996;12:64–9.
34. Hanson TW, Varner KE. Technique tip: limiting fluid extravasation into soft tissues during ankle arthroscopy before lateral ankle ligamentous reconstruction. Foot Ankle Int 2007;28:739–41.
35. Mercer D, Morrell NT, Fitzpatrick J, et al. The course of the distal saphenous nerve: a cadaveric investigation and clinical implications. Iowa Orthop J 2011; 31:231–5.
36. Prakash, Bhardwaj AK, Singh DK, et al. Anatomic variations of superficial peroneal nerve: clinical implications of a cadaver study. Ital J Anat Embryol 2010; 115:223–8.
37. de Leeuw PA, Golanó P, Sierevelt IN, et al. The course of the superficial peroneal nerve in relation to the ankle position: anatomical study with ankle arthroscopic implications. Knee Surg Sports Traumatol Arthrosc 2010;18:612–7.
38. Son KH, Cho JH, Lee JW, et al. Is the anterior tibial artery safe during ankle arthroscopy?: anatomic analysis of the anterior tibial artery at the ankle joint by magnetic resonance imaging. Am J Sports Med 2011;39:2452–6.
39. Deng DF, Hamilton GA, Lee M, et al. Complications associated with foot and ankle arthroscopy. J Foot Ankle Surg 2012;51:281–4.
40. Jacobs E, Groot D, Das M, et al. Pseudoaneurysm of the anterior tibial artery after ankle arthroscopy. J Foot Ankle Surg 2011;50:361–3.
41. Needleman RL. Fluoroscopic method for localization of the anteromedial portal for use in ankle arthroscopy: technique tip. J Foot Ankle Surg 2013;52:257–9.

42. Kelberine F, Frank A. Arthroscopic treatment of osteochondral lesions of the talar dome: a retrospective study of 48 cases. Arthroscopy 1999;15:77–84.
43. Hunt SA, Sherman O. Arthroscopic treatment of osteochondral lesions of the talus with correlation of outcome scoring systems. Arthroscopy 2003;19:360–7.
44. Wajsfisz A, Makridis KG, Naji O, et al. An anterior ankle arthroscopic technique for retrograde osteochondral autograft transplantation of posteromedial and central talar dome cartilage defects. Knee Surg Sports Traumatol Arthrosc 2014;22: 1298–303.
45. van Bergen CJ, Tuijthof GJ, Mass M, et al. Arthroscopic accessibility of the talus quantified by computed tomography simulation. Am J Sports Med 2012;40: 2318–24.
46. Ferkel RD, Scranton PE Jr, Stone JW, et al. Surgical treatment of osteochondral lesions of the talus. Instr Course Lect 2010;59:387–404.
47. van Dijk CN, van Bergen CJ. Advancements in ankle arthroscopy. J Am Acad Orthop Surg 2008;16:635–46.
48. Ferkel RD, Small HN, Gittins JE. Complications in foot and ankle arthroscopy. Clin Orthop Relat Res 2001;(391):89–104.
49. Simonson DC, Roukis TS. Safety of ankle arthroscopy for the treatment of anterolateral soft-tissue impingement. Arthroscopy 2014;30:256–9.
50. Ucerler H, Ikiz AA, Uygur M. A cadaver study on preserving peroneal nerves during ankle arthroscopy. Foot Ankle Int 2007;28:1172–8.
51. Solomon LB, Ferris L, Henneberg M. Anatomical study of the ankle with view to the anterior arthroscopic portals. ANZ J Surg 2006;76:932–6.
52. Suzangar M, Rosenfeld P. Ankle arthroscopy: is preoperative marking of the superficial peroneal nerve important? J Foot Ankle Surg 2012;51:179–81.
53. Ferkel RD, Heath DD, Guhl JF. Neurological complications of ankle arthroscopy. Arthroscopy 1996;12:200–8.
54. Kashir A, Kiely P, Dar W, et al. Pseudoaneurysm of the dorsalis pedis artery after ankle arthroscopy. Foot Ankle Surg 2010;16:151–2.
55. Jeffery CA, Quinn SJ, Quinn JM. Pseudoaneurysm of the anterior tibial artery after ankle arthroscopy. ANZ J Surg 2014;84:391–3.
56. Verbrugghe P, Vandekerkhof J, Baeyens I. Pseudoaneurysm of the anterior tibial artery: a complication of ankle arthroscopy. Acta Chir Belg 2011;111:410–1.
57. Brimmo OA, Parekh SG. Pseudoaneurysm as a complication of ankle arthroscopy. Indian J Orthop 2010;44:108–11.
58. Ramavath AL, Cornish JA, Ganapathi M, et al. Missed diagnosis of ankle pseudoaneurysm following ankle arthroscopy: a case report. Cases J 2009;2:162.
59. Vazquez T, Rodríguez-Niedenfuhr M, Parkin I, et al. Anatomic study of blood supply of the dorsum of the foot and ankle. Arthroscopy 2006;22:287–90.
60. Salzler MJ, Lin A, Miller CD, et al. Complications after arthroscopic knee surgery. Am J Sports Med 2014;42:292–6.
61. Greene JW, Deshmukh AJ, Cushner FD. Thromboembolic complications in arthroscopic surgery. Sports Med Arthrosc 2013;21:69–74.
62. Schade VL, Roukis TS. Antithrombotic pharmacologic prophylaxis use during conservative and surgical management of foot and ankle disorders: a systematic review. Clin Podiatr Med Surg 2011;28:571–88.
63. Rasmussen S, Hjorth Jensen C. Arthroscopic treatment of impingement of the ankle reduces pain and enhances function. Scand J Med Sci Sports 2002;12: 69–72.
64. Navadgi BC, Shah N, Jeer PJ. Rupture of the extensor hallucis longus tendon after ankle arthroscopy - an unusual complication. Foot Ankle Surg 2007;13:45–7.

65. Tuncer S, Aksu N, Isiklar U. Delayed rupture of the extensor hallucis longus and extensor digitorum communis tendons after breaching the anterior capsule with a radiofrequency probe during ankle arthroscopy: a case report. J Foot Ankle Surg 2010;49:490.e1–3.
66. Schmidt RG, Reddy CS. An unusual complication of an ankle arthroscopy and its management. J Foot Ankle Surg 1999;38:147–9.
67. Parma A, Buda R, Vannini F, et al. Arthroscopic treatment of ankle anterior bony impingement: the long-term clinical outcome. Foot Ankle Int 2014;35:148–55.

Ankle Instability and Arthroscopic Lateral Ligament Repair

Jorge I. Acevedo, MD[a],*, Peter Mangone, MD[b]

KEYWORDS

- Ankle instability • Arthroscopy • Arthroscopic lateral ankle ligament reconstruction
- Brostrom • Ankle sprain • All inside arthroscopic repair

KEY POINTS

- There is increasing interest in arthroscopic techniques to surgically correct chronic lateral ankle ligament instability.
- The anatomic "safe zone" in the lateral ankle allows surgeons to perform arthroscopic techniques safely.
- Recent published clinical and biomechanical studies show arthroscopic lateral ankle ligament reconstruction to have results similar to open modified Brostrom techniques.

INTRODUCTION

Ankle sprains are one of the most common lower extremity injuries.[1,2] Although most people recover without significant long-term consequences, chronic ankle instability does develop in about 20% of patients. Affected individuals usually complain of recurrent ankle sprains, difficulty with ambulation on uneven ground, and, in some cases, pain with activity.[1,3,4] Patients with cavovarus foot deformity, tibia vara, peroneal tendon injuries, and hyperligamentous laxity syndrome are at increased risk of chronic ankle instability.[1,5,6]

The normal treatment of a patient with chronic ankle instability focuses on a combination of peroneal muscle strengthening, balance reflex training, and external bracing as needed to prevent recurrent injury. Oftentimes, patients who follow these nonoperative regimens can successfully manage their instability without surgery.[1,7,8] Patients who fail these measures are candidates for lateral ankle ligament reconstruction.

Dr. Jorge I. Acevedo and Dr. Peter Mangone are the consultants for Arthrex Inc.
[a] Southeast Orthopedic Specialists, Jacksonville, 2627 Riverside Avenue, suite 300, FL 32204, USA; [b] Foot and Ankle Services, Foot and Ankle Center, Blue Ridge Bone and Joint Clinic, Mission Hospital, 60 Livingston Street, Asheville, NC 28801, USA
* Corresponding author.
E-mail address: ace4foot@gmail.com

Foot Ankle Clin N Am 20 (2015) 59–69
http://dx.doi.org/10.1016/j.fcl.2014.10.002
1083-7515/15/$ – see front matter © 2015 Elsevier Inc. All rights reserved.

Traditionally, the primary surgical treatment performed is the Brostrom or augmented Brostrom technique using either drill holes or the more contemporary suture anchor techniques.[1,7,9,10] More complex tendon reconstructive techniques are normally reserved for either failed primary reconstructions or patients at high risk for failure with a primary Brostrom-Gould technique.[1,6,11,12]

Over the last 40 years, there has been an evolution in the surgical treatment of instability in the knee and shoulder. Initially procedures were performed in an open manner with nonanatomic methods externally to restrain abnormal motion. This method was then followed by arthroscopic examination followed by open procedures. Subsequently, surgeons moved toward arthroscopic examination with mini-open procedures. Finally, fully arthroscopic stabilization procedures have become the current standard of care in the knee and the shoulder.[13-15]

The concept of minimally invasive lateral ankle ligament reconstruction was first introduced in the use of a mini-open technique and stapling to the fibula.[16] Although fully arthroscopic procedures for knee and shoulder instability have advanced significantly since then, the concept of arthroscopic lateral ankle ligament reconstruction has been slow to move forward until recently. In the last 5 years, there has been significantly increased interest in arthroscopic techniques to address chronic lateral ankle instability.

In this review, the authors begin with a discussion of the anatomy and biomechanics of the lateral ankle ligament complex. The pertinent anatomy and biomechanics related to arthroscopic lateral ankle ligament reconstruction is then explored. Publications of recent clinical studies using arthroscopic techniques are reviewed. Finally, the intraoperative technique proven to be biomechanically equivalent to the current open Brostrom technique and most familiar to the authors is described.

ANATOMY AND BIOMECHANICS

Understanding the anatomy of the lateral ligamentous complex is essential to the diagnosis and treatment of ankle instability. When considering arthroscopic lateral ligament repair it is equally important to have proper anatomic knowledge of the structures surrounding this complex. To simplify this section, the authors first discuss the basic ligament anatomy and its relation to lateral ankle instability, and then describe the anatomy as it relates to the arthroscopic ligament repair.

Lateral Ligamentous Complex and Biomechanics of the Normal Lateral Ankle

The lateral ligamentous support of the ankle comprises 3 main structures: the anterior talofibular ligament (ATFL), the calcaneofibular ligament (CFL), and the posterior talofibular ligament (PTFL). The ATFL is the most frequently injured ligament with inversion sprains.[17,18] Most commonly, it consists of 2 bands originating at the anterior margin of the distal fibula with the center averaging 10 mm from the tip of the lateral malleolus.[19-21] From the origin, it runs anteromedially to a bifid insertion on the body of the talus anterior to the articular margin.[20,22] The ATFL is the weakest of the lateral ankle ligaments (ultimate failure, load 138–160 N) and thus most prone to injury with inversion sprains.[23]

The CFL originates as a confluent footprint with the ATFL on the anterior border of the distal fibula. It then courses deep to the peroneal tendons to insert on a tubercle on the lateral wall of the calcaneus. This footprint lays approximately 3 cm posterior and superior to the peroneal tubercle.[20] Although combined rupture may occur in up to 20% of cases, clinical and biomechanical studies have not demonstrated direct repair of this ligament to be essential to good outcomes.[9,24-26]

The PTFL arises from the medial surface of the lateral malleolus and inserts in a multifasicular fashion along the posterolateral talus.[22] Some fibers may even course proximally to render a tibial slip. Because this ligament is relaxed in plantarflexion, it is unlikely to be a major contributor to stability in the typical inversion sprain but may be involved in posterior ankle impingement syndromes.

The subtalar joint ligaments may also play a role in ankle instability but are not as well described. The inferior extensor retinaculum (IER), the lateral talocalcaneal ligament, the cervical ligament, and the interosseous talocalcaneal ligament have all been implicated in providing subtalar joint stability.[5,20] Although it is widely accepted that these ligaments may be injured in conjunction with the lateral ligament complex, the exact mechanism is not well understood. Their importance, as it relates to the arthroscopic lateral ligament repair, may be related to the inclusion of the IER in the ArthroBrostrom procedure. Because of the calcaneal attachments of the IER, the authors believe this ligament imparts further stability to the repair.[27,28]

Arthroscopic Ligament Repair Anatomy

When performing an arthroscopic lateral ligament repair, it is important to have a good understanding of the proximity of the surrounding structures. There is a paucity of anatomic studies defining the safe zones and structures at risk for the arthroscopic repair. Drakos and colleagues[29] examined the superficial and deep anatomy of the lateral ankle after arthroscopic repair of the lateral ligament complex. Results from this study showed a high risk of entrapment (9 of 55 structures) of the extensor tendons and superficial peroneal nerve (SPN). Actual entrapment of the nerve occurred in 2 of the 5 specimens in which the intermediate branch of the SPN was identified. The arthroscopic procedure used in this study required an accessory portal and attempted to repair the CFL, which may have increased the incidence of entrapment. The authors do not believe repair of the CFL is necessary and therefore do not incorporate this into the ArthroBrostrom procedure previously described.[27,28] This procedure is consistent with a recent study by Lee and colleagues[25] showing long-term excellent results with an open technique in which the CFL was not repaired; instead, attention was focused on a combined reconstruction of the ATFL, capsule, and IER.

One of the authors (JIA) evaluated the safe zones for the proximity of anatomic structures for the ArthroBrostrom lateral ankle ligament stabilization and defined the ideal landmarks and safe zone for this repair.[27] The study revealed no incidence of nerve entrapment with a mean safe distance of 20 mm (range, 8–36 mm) between the medial suture knot and the SPN. An even safer mean distance of 23 mm (range, 17–35 mm) was measured from the inferior suture knot to the sural nerve. An internervous safe zone of a mean 51 mm was identified between the SPN and sural nerves. Similarly, an intertendinous safe zone of a mean 43 mm between the peroneus tertius and peroneus brevis tendons was located. When the ankle was placed in neutral dorsiflexion, sufficient portions of the IER were grasped if sutures were passed at an average 15 mm from the tip of the fibula. Because the ArthroBrostrom procedure does not repair the CFL, the authors recommend passage of sutures through the IER to improve subtalar stability.

Biomechanics of Arthroscopic Lateral Ankle Ligament Reconstruction

There are several biomechanical studies published examining the Brostrom, modified Brostrom, and tendon transfer/allograft techniques.[23,30–34] Despite all efforts to recreate normal anatomy, recent published data have shown open techniques still remain inferior to the native ATFL uninjured tissue.[23,34]

Although publications detailed in the clinical section of this review have highlighted the clinical success using arthroscopic lateral ankle ligament reconstruction techniques, biomechanical data have been limited until recently. Both Dracos and colleagues[35] in 2011 and Giza and colleagues[36] in 2013 published data revealing biomechanically equivalent results of arthroscopic versus open techniques when using matched cadaver pairs. Dracos's technique used 2 anchors, with 1 anchor inserted in the inferior fibula through an accessory portal.[35] Giza's research used the ArthroBrostrom all-inside technique using the typical standard anteromedial and anterolateral arthroscopic portals.[36]

Although these studies are compelling, additional studies are needed to prove the best technique to try and reconstruct incompetent lateral ankle ligaments.

CLINICAL RESULTS

Most lateral ligament injuries can be treated nonsurgically, but up to 20% of patients will develop chronic recurrent instability resulting from sensory-motor deficits or insufficient healing of the lateral ligament complex.[1,3,4,37–39] Operative treatment is indicated for those patients with a history of multiple inversion events and continued episodes of instability despite conservative treatment.[39] The open modified Brostrom-Gould anatomic repair has been widely accepted as the standard technique for lateral ankle stabilization. In the classic Brostrom-Gould technique, both the calcaneofibular and the anterior talofibular ligaments are repaired with subsequent reinforcement with the IER.[1] Several different nonanatomic techniques have been reported in the literature with similar long-term results but with increased morbidity.[1,3,40,41] Owing to the potential for overtightening from augmented procedures, the Brostrom-Gould remains the technique of choice for most surgeons when performing a primary lateral ankle stabilization.[11,25,41,42]

Since the first report in 1987, arthroscopic ankle stabilization has been emerging as a viable alternative to open techniques. Hawkins initially described an arthroscopic technique using staples for plication of the lateral ankle ligaments.[16] This procedure required 2 additional portals as well as an abrasion of the lateral talar surface. Results in 24 patients were promising with only one recurrence, and most of the complications were due to staple prominence. Subsequently, the first arthroscopic technique using suture anchors to repair the lateral ligamentous complex was proposed by Kashuk.[43] The investigators used one additional accessory anterolateral portal to place the suture anchors, which necessitated penetrating through the lateral ankle ligaments. Unfortunately, no outcomes analysis was performed in this study.[28]

After these initial reports of arthroscopic stabilization, arthroscopic thermal capsular shrinkage was adapted for use in the ankle because of its initial success for instability in other joints. Despite failures for the treatment of shoulder and knee instability, thermal shrinkage may be more effective in the chronically unstable ankle because of the intrinsic stability of the ankle mortise. Initial series implemented this technique for mild or functional ankle instability with 80% to 86% good to excellent results.[10,44] More recent studies extending indications to mechanical instability have rendered less favorable results.[45] As a result, there has been a resurgence of interest in arthroscopic techniques that have attempted to maintain the minimally invasive approach while providing the stability of the traditional open Brostrom-Gould procedure.

Several clinical studies have reported favorable outcomes for patients treated with the arthroscopic-assisted repairs.[27,46–48] In 2009, Corte-Real and Moreira[46] reported the first European study on 28 of their 31 patients using an arthroscopic-assisted technique. The investigators used one double-loaded suture anchor as well as an accessory anterolateral portal. At 24.5-month average follow-up, American Orthopedic Foot and Ankle Society (AOFAS) scores averaged 85.3 and only 2 patients demonstrated recurrent instability.SPN injury occurred in 3 cases, but only 1 persisted. Kim and colleagues[47] subsequently published their results on 28 ankles also using 1 double-loaded suture anchor. Unlike the prior technique, these investigators used a soft-tissue penetrator to pass sutures and used an accessory anteroinferior portal. At a 15.9-month average follow-up, 3 patients had laxity with stress radiographs but all were able to return to their preinjury level. The longest follow-up study to date was reported by Nery and colleagues[48] on 38 patients with an average 9.8-year follow-up. Their technique also used 1 double-loaded anchor into the anterior fibula and an accessory portal to lasso the ligamentous complex. The mean AOFAS score was 90%, and 87% of active patients continued to practice sport at the same preoperative level 10 years after the repair.

Several studies have described an all-inside arthroscopic ligament technique with good outcomes.[28,49,50] The authors reported their initial series of 24 ankles performed from 2007 to 2011 with no known recurrences. At a mean 16.5-month follow-up AOFAS scores improved from 54 to 92. This technique simplifies all prior methods so that only the 2 standard anterior portals are necessary. The procedure allows for placement of 2 individual suture anchors, which the authors believe improves stability and pull-out strength. Separate passes of the sutures engage a wider surface area and may potentially avoid inadvertent injury to the SPN.[28] Cottom and Rigby[49] reported results using the same technique on 40 patients with a mean 1-year follow-up. AOFAS scores improved from 41 to 95 and clinical assessment demonstrated excellent stability of the lateral ankle ligaments and negative anterior drawer test at the final follow-up visit.

Vega and colleagues[50] described a modified all-inside technique whereby a nitinol looped suture passer is used to pass a doubled suture through the ATFL. Although an accessory portal is necessary, the method implements a knotless suture anchor and therefore avoids the potential complication of knot prominence. At a mean follow-up of 22.3 months, all 16 patients reported subjective improvement of their ankle instability with an AOFAS mean score of 97 and no complications. Potential disadvantages of this pure anatomic technique are that neither the CFL nor the IER is repaired.

The authors have reviewed their latest follow-up of 93 patients who have undergone the ArthroBrostrom procedure from November 2007. At this time there are adequate preoperative and postoperative data for review on 73 patients. Although many of the 20 patients for whom the authors are missing data are doing well, their data are currently incomplete; therefore, the authors have decided to exclude their results at this time. Average age was 35 years, with a 2:1 female to male ratio. Mean follow-up was 28 months. Karlsson-Peterson scores improved substantially from a preoperative mean of 28.3 to a postoperative mean of 90.2. Only 1 patient had recurrent instability. Of 73 patients, 69 were satisfied with the results. Four patients were dissatisfied. Of the dissatisfied patients, 1 had recurrent instability and 3 had persistent pain symptoms postoperatively. Of those failures, 2 of 4 failures were workman's compensation patients. Five patients developed postoperative neuritis, with 1 patient's symptoms resolving after removal of the sutures that had entrapped the intermediate branch of the SPN.

ARTHROBROSTROM INTRAOPERATIVE TECHNIQUE

Although there are several different published arthroscopic techniques for lateral ankle ligament reconstruction, this review discusses the technique the authors helped develop, which has proven biomechanical equivalency to the open Brostrom-Gould procedure.

- Anesthesia: Most patients can have a regional popliteal block plus monitored anesthesia care (MAC). Some patients may require a general anesthesia. If a regional popliteal block is performed, the surgeon or anesthesiologist usually must perform a separate local block for the saphenous nerve to cover the anteromedial portal.
- Distraction versus no distraction: The arthroscopy and arthroscopic lateral ligament reconstruction can be performed with either method. The surgeon should use his/her preference. It is important to remember that if distraction is used, the distraction is removed before tying the sutures to tighten the lateral ankle ligament complex.
- Preoperative drawing of anatomic landmarks: This step is critical for success and involves marking the safe zone in the lateral ankle region.[27,46] The peroneal tendons, distal fibula, and intermediate branch of the SPN are identified and outlined on the skin. The location of the IER is estimated and drawn using the lateral calcaneal tubercle to help identify the margin of this tissue (**Fig. 1**).
- Standard anteromedial and anterolateral arthroscopy portals are used.
- Normal diagnostic arthroscopy is performed and any additional intra-articular pathology that exists is addressed in the normal manner before the ligament procedure. The surgeon must perform a more extensive debridement of the lateral gutter for 2 purposes: to reduce impingement/clean out the pathologic fibrotic tissue that usually fills the lateral gutter and to allow for adequate visualization of the anterior distal face of the fibula for proper placement and passage of the sutures.
- The inferior tip of the fibula is identified with a probe.
- Using the standard anterolateral portal, the first bone anchor is then placed 1 cm superior to the tip of the fibula, with the sutures being brought out of the standard anterolateral portal. This first set of sutures is then passed one at a time using a sharp tipped suture passer. This step can be performed with either an inside-out technique or an outside-in technique. Care is taken to make sure the exit point is at least 2 cm distal to the anterior face of the fibula to ensure capture of the IER.[27,35] This method is performed while viewing from the anteromedial portal.
  - First set of sutures: The first suture is passed just superior to the peroneal tendons, and the second suture is passed 1 cm dorsal/anterior to the first suture along the arc of the IER.

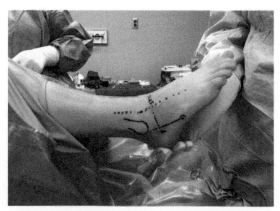

Fig. 1. Landmarks drawn to establish the anatomic safe zone before beginning the arthroscopy.

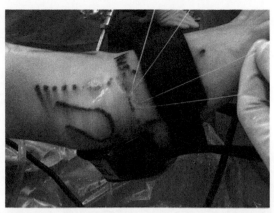

Fig. 2. Photograph taken after both sets of sutures have been passed using a sharp-tipped curved suture passer. The next step is to make a small incision between the sets of sutures to allow for passage and tying.

- The second anchor is then placed 1 cm superior to the first anchor in the anterior face of the fibula. This point should still be located inferior to the level of the talar dome as the ATFL anatomic origin is inferior the talar dome. The second set of sutures is then passed with a sharp-tipped suture passer while visualized through the anteromedial portal.
  - Second set of sutures: The first suture is passed about 1 cm dorsal/anterior to the last suture from the first anchor along the arc of the IER. The second suture from the second anchor is then passed through the tissue 1 cm dorsal/anterior form the first suture. Care is taken to make sure the second suture stays inferior to the intermediate branch of the SPN in the safe zone (**Fig. 2**).
- A small incision is then made between the 2 sets of sutures, and using a small arthroscopic hook, the suture sets are then passed through this central incision. If the surgeon is concerned about the intermediate branch of the SPN, he/she can simply retract the tissue anteriorly through the incision to make sure the more superior set of sutures has been passed deep to the nerve to prevent entrapment (**Fig. 3**).

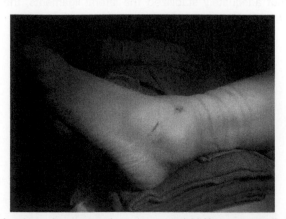

Fig. 3. Photograph taken after sutures have been tied (different patient). The standard anterolateral arthroscopy portal can be seen as well as the small oblique incision made to pass and tie the sutures to imbricate the capsule, anterior talofibular ligament, and inferior extensor retinaculum.

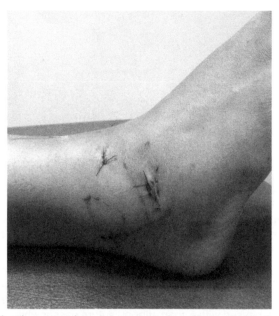

Fig. 4. Photograph taken 1 week post-op. Minimal swelling present. One can still see the residual ink on the skin from marking the anatomic landmarks to establish the safe zone and location of the inferior extensor retinaculum.

- The ankle is then held in neutral to slight eversion at 90° with a slight posterior drawer pressure. The sutures are then tied down over the capsule and IER causing these to imbricate and pull up to the face of the anterior fibula when viewed through the arthroscope.
- The construct is tested for stability. If the surgeon prefers, he/she can add to the construct with supplemental suture techniques such as a suture bridge or internal brace-type construct. Should the surgeon decide that the arthroscopic technique has not adequately stabilized the lateral ligaments, the procedure can easily be converted to an open technique at any point.

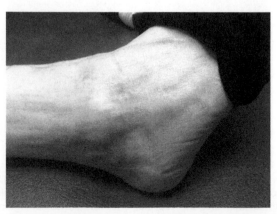

Fig. 5. Photograph taken 6 months post-op. Incisional scars are barely visible.

- If the surgeon is concerned about a possible peroneal tendon tear, a small incision can be made directly over the peroneal tendons to examine and perform a repair as necessary. Alternatively, the surgeon could perform a peroneal tendonoscopy to examine the anatomy.
- The arthroscopic portals and the small incision for suture tying are then closed with a small nylon mattress suture (**Fig. 4**).
- With the smaller incisions and less soft-tissue dissection, immediate postoperative swelling is far less than normal and the long-term cosmetic appearance is excellent (**Fig. 5**).

SUMMARY

The goal of any arthroscopic procedure is to replace traditional open techniques while obtaining results that are at least equivalent, if not better, than current operative techniques and patient outcomes. Shoulder and knee orthopedic specialists have successfully converted to arthroscopic techniques to deal with most chronic instability patients; however, foot and ankle orthopedists have been previously reluctant to move in the same direction. Multiple studies that reveal both clinical and biomechanical equivalent results between traditional open modified Brostrom ligament reconstruction and newer arthroscopic lateral ankle ligament reconstruction techniques have now been completed. Although additional studies need to be performed and published, the authors believe evidence is mounting that arthroscopic lateral ankle ligament reconstruction is a reasonable and viable alternative to traditional open techniques and should be considered as a potential alternative to traditional open techniques.

REFERENCES

1. Colville M. Surgical treatment of the unstable ankle. J Am Acad Orthop Surg 1998;6:368–77.
2. Colville MR, Marder RA, Zarins B. Reconstruction of the lateral ankle ligaments: a biomechanical analysis. Am J Sports Med 1992;20:594–600.
3. Chan KW, Ding BC, Mroczek KJ. Acute and chronic lateral ankle instability in the athlete. Bull NYU Hosp Jt Dis 2011;69(1):17–26.
4. Freeman MA. Instability of the foot after injuries to the lateral ligament of the ankle. J Bone Joint Surg Br 1965;47(4):669–77.
5. Karlsson J, Eriksson BI, Renstrom P. Subtalar joint instability of the foot: a review and results after surgical treatment. Scand J Med Sci Sports 1998;8:191–7.
6. Schindler OS. Surgery for anterior cruciate ligament deficiency: a historical perspective. Knee Surg Sports Traumatol Arthrosc 2012;20(1):5–47.
7. Ringleb SI, Dhakal A, Anderson CD, et al. Effects of lateral ligament sectioning on the stability of the ankle and subtalar joint. J Orthop Res 2011;29(10):1459–64.
8. Sammarco GJ, Carrasquillo HA. Surgical revision after failed lateral ankle reconstruction. Foot Ankle Int 1995;16(12):748–53.
9. Broström L. Sprained ankles. VI. Surgical treatment of "chronic" ligament ruptures. Acta Chir Scand 1966;132(5):551–65.
10. Maiotti M, Massoni C, Tarantino U. The use of arthroscopic thermal shrinkage to treat chronic lateral ankle instability in young athletes. Arthroscopy 2005;21(6):751–7.
11. Hennrikus WL, Mapes RC, Lyons PM, et al. Outcomes of the Chrisman-Snook and modified Broström procedure for chronic lateral ankle instability. A prospective, randomized comparison. Am J Sports Med 1996;24:400–4.

12. Sammarco GJ, Idusuyi OB. Reconstruction of the lateral ankle ligaments using a split peroneus brevis tendon graft. Foot Ankle Int 1999;20(2):97–103.
13. Godin J, Sekiya JK. Systematic review of arthroscopic versus open repair for recurrent anterior shoulder dislocations. Sports Health 2011;3(4):396–404.
14. Sedeek S, Gerard E, Andrew H. Evolution of arthroscopic shoulder stabilization: do we still need open techniques? OA Orthopaedics 2013;1(1):1.
15. Strauss JE, Forsberg JA, Lippert FG. Chronic lateral ankle instability and associated conditions: a rationale for treatment. Foot Ankle Int 2007;28(10):1041–4.
16. Hawkins RB. Arthroscopic stapling repair for chronic lateral instability. Clin Podiatr Med Surg 1987;4(4):875–83.
17. Boruta PM, Bishop JO, Braly WG, et al. Acute lateral ankle ligament injuries: a literature review. Foot Ankle 1990;11(2):107–13.
18. Hintermann B. Biomechanics of the unstable ankle joint and clinical implications. Med Sci Sports Exerc 1999;31(7 Suppl):S459–69.
19. Burks RT, Morgan J. Anatomy of the lateral ankle ligaments. Am J Sports Med 1994;22:72–7.
20. Neuschwander TB, Indresano AA, Hughes TH, et al. Footprint of the lateral ligament complex of the ankle. Foot Ankle Int 2013;34(4):582–6.
21. Pihlajamäki H, Hietaniemi K, Paavola M, et al. Surgical versus functional treatment for acute ruptures of the lateral ligament complex of the ankle in young men: a randomized controlled trial. J Bone Joint Surg Am 2010;92(14):2367–74.
22. Golanó P, Vega J, De leeuw PA, et al. Anatomy of the ankle ligaments: a pictorial essay. Knee Surg Sports Traumatol Arthrosc 2010;18(5):557–69.
23. Viens NA, Wijdicks CA, Campbell KJ, et al. Anterior talofibular ligament ruptures, part 1: biomechanical comparison of augmented Broström repair techniques with the intact anterior talofibular ligament. Am J Sports Med 2014;42(2):405–11.
24. Lee KT, Lee JI, Sung KS, et al. Biomechanical evaluation against calcaneofibular ligament repair in the Brostrom procedure: a cadaveric study. Knee Surg Sports Traumatol Arthrosc 2008;16(8):781–6.
25. Lee KT, Park YU, Kim JS, et al. Long-term results after modified Brostrom procedure without calcaneofibular ligament reconstruction. Foot Ankle Int 2011;32(2):153–7.
26. Li X, Killie H, Guerrero P, et al. Anatomical reconstruction for chronic lateral ankle instability in the high-demand athlete: functional outcomes after the modified Broström repair using suture anchors. Am J Sports Med 2009;37(3):488–94.
27. Acevedo JI. ArthroBrostrom lateral ankle stabilization technique: an anatomical study. Paper presented at: AANA 2014. Proceedings of the 33rd Annual Meeting of the Arthroscopy Association of North America. Hollywood (FL), May 1–3, 2014.
28. Acevedo JI, Mangone PG. Arthroscopic lateral ankle ligament reconstruction. Tech Foot Ankle Surg 2011;10(3):111–6.
29. Drakos M, Behrens SB, Mulcahey MK, et al. Proximity of arthroscopic ankle stabilization procedures to surrounding structures: an anatomic study. Arthroscopy 2013;29(6):1089–94.
30. Clanton TO, Viens NA, Campbell KJ, et al. Anterior talofibular ligament ruptures, part 2: biomechanical comparison of anterior talofibular ligament reconstruction using semitendinosus allografts with the intact ligament. Am J Sports Med 2014;42(2):412–6.
31. Fujii T, Kitaoka HB, Watanabe K, et al. Comparison of modified Broström and Evans procedures in simulated lateral ankle injury. Med Sci Sports Exerc 2006;38(6):1025–31.

32. Hollis JM, Blasier RD, Flahiff CM, et al. Biomechanical comparison of reconstruction techniques in simulated lateral ankle ligament injury. Am J Sports Med 1995; 23(6):678–82.
33. Wainright WB, Spritzer CE, Lee JY, et al. The effect of modified Broström-Gould repair for lateral ankle instability on in vivo tibiotalar kinematics. Am J Sports Med 2012;40(9):2099–104.
34. Waldrop NE 3rd, Wijdicks CA, Jansson KS, et al. Anatomic suture anchor versus the Brostrom technique for anterior talofibular ligament repair: a biomechanical comparison. Am J Sports Med 2012;40(11):2590–6.
35. Drakos M, Behrens S, Hoffman E, et al. A biomechanical comparison of an open vs. arthroscopic approach for the treatment of lateral ankle instability (SS-57). Arthroscopy 2011;27(5).
36. Giza E, Shin EC, Wong SE, et al. Arthroscopic suture anchor repair of the lateral ligament ankle complex: a cadaveric study. Am J Sports Med 2013;41(11): 2567–72.
37. de Vries JS, Krips R, Sierevelt IN, et al. Interventions for treating chronic ankle instability. Cochrane Database Syst Rev 2011;(8):CD004124.
38. Gerber JP, Williams GN, Scoville CR, et al. Persistent disability associated with ankle sprains: a prospective examination of an athletic population. Foot Ankle Int 1998;19:653–60.
39. Karlsson J, Bergsten T, Lansinger O, et al. Reconstruction of the lateral ligaments of the ankle for chronic lateral instability. J Bone Joint Surg Am 1988;70(4):581–8.
40. Becker HP, Ebner S, Ebner D, et al. 12-year outcome after modified Watson-Jones tenodesis for ankle instability. Clin Orthop Relat Res 1999;(358):194–204.
41. Miller AG, Raikin SM, Ahmad J. Near-anatomic allograft tenodesis of chronic lateral ankle instability. Foot Ankle Int 2013;34(11):1501–7.
42. Bell SJ, Mologne TS, Sitler DF, et al. Twenty-six-year results after Brostrom procedure for chronic lateral ankle instability. Am J Sports Med 2006;34:975–8.
43. Kashuk KB, Landsman AS, Werd MB, et al. Arthroscopic lateral ankle stabilization. Clin Podiatr Med Surg 1994;11(3):407–23.
44. Berlet GC, Saar WE, Ryan A, et al. Thermal-assisted capsular modification for functional ankle instability. Foot Ankle Clin 2002;7(3):567–76.
45. de Vries JS, Krips R, Blankevoort L, et al. Arthroscopic capsular shrinkage for chronic ankle instability with thermal radiofrequency: prospective multicenter trial. Orthopedics 2008;31(7):655.
46. Corte-Real NM, Moreira RM. Arthroscopic repair of chronic lateral ankle instability. Foot Ankle Int 2009;30:213–7.
47. Kim ES, Lee KT, Park JS, et al. Arthroscopic anterior talofibular ligament repair for chronic ankle instability with a suture anchor technique. Orthopedics 2011;34(4): 1–5.
48. Nery C, Raduan F, Del Buono A, et al. Arthroscopic-assisted Brostrom-Gould for chronic ankle instability: a long-term follow-up. Am J Sports Med 2011;39(11): 2381–8.
49. Cottom JM, Rigby RB. The "all inside" arthroscopic Brostrom procedure: a prospective study of 40 consecutive patients. J Foot Ankle Surg 2013;52(5):568–74.
50. Vega J, Golanó P, Pellegrino A, et al. All-inside arthroscopic lateral collateral ligament repair for ankle instability with a knotless suture anchor technique. Foot Ankle Int 2013;34(12):1701–9.

Arthroscopic Ankle Arthrodesis

Anna O. Elmlund, PhD, Ian G. Winson, FRCS*

KEYWORDS

- Arthroscopic • Ankle • Tibiotalar • Arthrodesis • Fusion

KEY POINTS

- Arthroscopic ankle arthrodesis is a good option for the treatment of end-stage ankle arthritis.
- Joint surfaces, except the lateral gutter, are prepared to point bleeding with motorized burr, abraider, and curettes.
- Standard anteromedial and anterolateral portals are used for ankle arthroscopy.

 Videos of joint preparation and excision of anterior osteophytes accompany this article at http://www.foot.theclinics.com/

INTRODUCTION: NATURE OF THE PROBLEM

Ankle arthrodesis is a well-established technique in the treatment of ankle arthritis.

The alternative of ankle replacement is not an option for all patients and has higher complication and revision rates.[1]

Although open arthrodesis has long been used with a variety of techniques, it is recognized as having a significant complication rate for both infection and nonunion.

With increasing pressure on reducing hospital stays and improving speed and reliability of overall recovery, arthroscopic arthrodesis has emerged as a viable option. Arthroscopic ankle fusions require shorter hospital stays, demonstrate quicker time to union with equivalent or higher union rates, exhibit faster recovery and possibly shorter operation time,[2,3] and ultimately lower costs.[4]

This article reviews both the technique and the reported results for arthroscopic ankle arthrodesis (AAA).

INDICATIONS/CONTRAINDICATIONS

The indications for AAA surgery include all the causes of end-stage ankle arthritis. It is particularly useful in cases in which there is soft tissue compromise surrounding the ankle joint.

The authors have nothing to disclose.
Avon Orthopaedic Centre, Southmead Hospital, Westbury-on-Trym, Bristol BS10 5NB, UK
* Corresponding author.
E-mail address: ianwinson@doctors.org.uk

When the potential causes of ankle arthritis are considered, the soft tissues and their management become a significant consideration. Posttraumatic arthritis frequently results in patients who have had the most severe types of trauma; this can include open cases and cases in which operative treatment has led to multiple scars.

Most series on ankle arthritis management have a relatively low average age (usually 45 years) and a high incidence of trauma (usually about 50%), and these trauma cases are exactly the sort of cases in which wound healing would be a potential problem with open techniques.

AAA is indicated in patients with inflammatory arthritis and in older patients in whom the problem of skin healing may be an issue. Limiting the required approach to stab incisions for arthroscopic portals and similarly small incisions for percutaneous screw fixation is desirable.

One of the contraindications to the arthroscopic technique is said to be deformity. The published literature would suggest otherwise.[5,6]

The key is whether the forefoot can be placed square to the ground.

The treating surgeon has to divide the deformity into deformity through the ankle where the preparation of the joint allows correction and deformity below the level of the joint where the foot position was effectively abnormal in the first place. The position of the ankle is only relevant to the position of the foot in which correction of the forefoot position and hindfoot position by suitable osteotomies would be necessary.

The presence of poor skin is only a relative contraindication as is the presence of metalwork from previous surgery. This condition may lead to a need to modify the technique to allow screw placement through healthy skin or in such a way that avoids metalwork.

Similarly, avascular necrosis of the talus is only a relative contraindication, and it can be argued that it is a relative indication for the arthroscopic technique if fusion is to be attempted.

Poor vascularity is a relative contraindication and should be analyzed as to its severity. But using an arthroscopic technique minimizes the risk of wound healing problems.

Although not an absolute contraindication, smoking is a factor that does increase the risk of nonunion irrespective of the approach.

Patients should be counseled to give up smoking and certainly should be advised that their risk of nonunion will be greatly increased.

The presence of neuropathy is again a relative contraindication. There is an increased risk of nonunion, and this is certainly true at an early stage of an active Charcot arthropathy.

The presence of active infection is an absolute contraindication.

SURGICAL TECHNIQUE/PROCEDURE
Preoperative Planning

When considering a patient for AAA, confirming that the symptoms are coming from the ankle is paramount.

Careful history taking and examination remains the best way of ensuring that the patient's symptoms are coming from the ankle as opposed to the other major joints.

Plain standing anteroposterior and lateral radiographs are useful (**Figs. 1** and **2**).

In addition, the use of a targeted injection of local anesthetic is a useful way of testing whether the pain is restricted to the ankle.

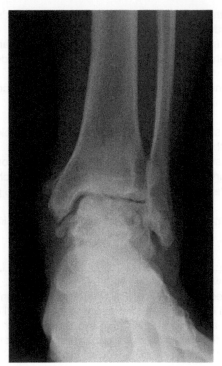

Fig. 1. Preoperative radiograph in standing position, frontal view.

Once the decision has been made to perform surgery, careful preparation is necessary.

Preparation and Patient Positioning

Preoperative prophylactic intravenous antibiotics, according to the local protocols, is recommended.

The routine use of general and/or regional anesthesia is required because full relaxation of the limb is necessary.

The patient is positioned supine on the operating table. A suitable-sized sandbag under ipsilateral buttock is used to maintain the position of the limb.

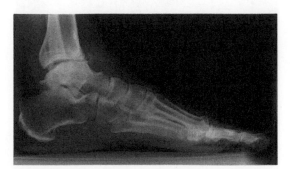

Fig. 2. Preoperative radiograph in standing position, lateral view.

A tourniquet on the thigh is inflated according to the surgeon's choice. It is possible to do the whole procedure without tourniquet.

The leg is prepared up to the knee. This is necessary to prepare the leg high enough to assess limb alignment and to have good access to place guidewires and screws for fixation (**Fig. 3**).

Traction with a noninvasive device is very useful but not necessary (see **Fig. 3**).

The surgical technique involves a standard 4.5- or 5.0-mm 30° scope ("kneescope").

Power instruments, such as a 4.5-mm full-radius arthroscopic shaver, can provide initial debridement of the joint, improving visualization.

Simple instruments such as curettes and even small osteotomes can be helpful in denuding the joint of articular cartilage and preparing the subchondral surface.

A motorized burr, preferably a barrel-shaped burr, is used to prepare the subchondral surfaces.

A system for cannulated compression screw fixation 6.5 mm in diameter or similar is necessary for fixation.

Surgical Approach

The joint is distended with an injection of 20 mL saline.

A standard anteromedial (medial to the tibialis anterior tendon) portal is used for the arthroscope, after skin incision and blunt dissection with small clip **Fig. 3**.

Under direct vision, an anterolateral (lateral to the extensor digitorum communis) portal is established in the same way. Care should be taken not to injure the lateral superficial peroneal nerve located subcutaneously **Fig. 3**.

Surgical Procedure

The remaining cartilage is removed with both curettes and a soft tissue resector (**Figs. 4–6**).

The joint surfaces are prepared with the burr from anterior to posterior to reveal healthy cancellous bone (**Figs. 7** and **8**, Videos 1–4).

If there are difficulties in reaching posteriorly, usually more bone needs to be resected anteriorly. Care must be taken to reduce the size of anterior osteophytes (see Video 2).

The lateral gutter needs to be cleared of osteophytes to allow reduction particularly in a varus ankle, but joint surfaces need not be prepared.

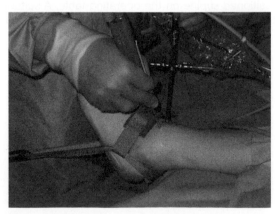

Fig. 3. Surgical position.

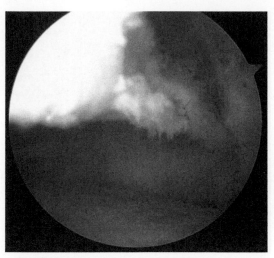

Fig. 4. Arthroscopic view before joint surface preparation, anterolateral view.

In contrast, the medial gutter is prepared thoroughly over the whole of the medial malleolus. The reciprocal surface of the medial facet of the talus should also be prepared (see Video 4).

Debris are removed with soft tissue resector.

Punctuate bleeding from bone can be demonstrated with maximal suction on the power instruments (see **Figs. 7** and **8**, Video 4).

The joint should be positioned in neutral flexion, 0°–5° hindfoot valgus, and a few degrees of external rotation compared with the contralateral side.

For standard fixation, 2 preferably parallel guide wires are inserted from the posteromedial side of the tibia through stab incisions.

Obtaining rigid fixation is the first priority; understanding compression is critical in obtaining an arthrodesis.

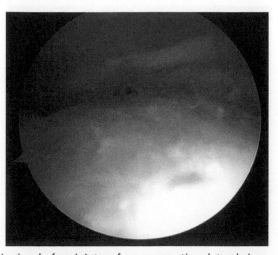

Fig. 5. Arthroscopic view before joint surface preparation, lateral view.

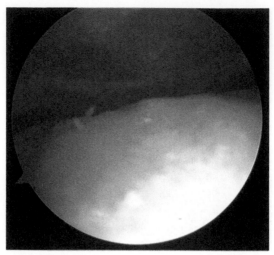

Fig. 6. Arthroscopic view before joint surface preparation, central view.

Fluoroscopic guidance is used throughout this phase of the surgery.
Care is taken not to penetrate into the subtalar joint.
Other screw constructs include a third screw, which provides further stability.
Compression screws of minimum 6.5 mm are inserted (**Figs. 9** and **10**).
Skin closure is usually performed with nonabsorbable sutures.

COMPLICATIONS AND MANAGEMENT

Complications include general surgical risks such as deep venous thrombosis/pulmonary embolism, which should be prevented according to the local protocol. The authors' favored method is to use mechanical means of prophylaxis. Anatomic structures at risk include the superficial peroneal nerve, located near the anterolateral

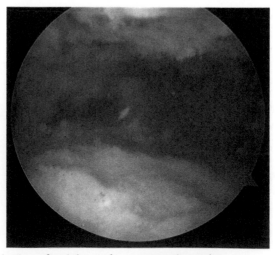

Fig. 7. Arthroscopic view after joint surface preparation, talus.

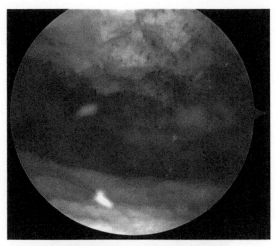

Fig. 8. Arthroscopic view after joint surface preparation, tibia.

portal, and the tibial nerve and posterior tibial artery, located at the posteromedial aspect of the ankle joint. Infections are reported, although the risk is lower with arthroscopic surgery. The literature suggests that the risk is about 1 in 500. First-line treatment would be antibiotics according to swab results and sensitivity with screws remaining in situ until bony fusion, when they can be removed. On the rare occasion

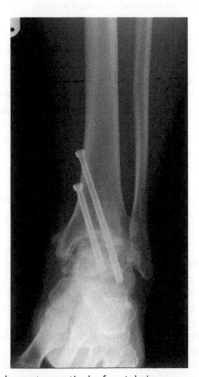

Fig. 9. Radiograph 12 weeks postoperatively, frontal view.

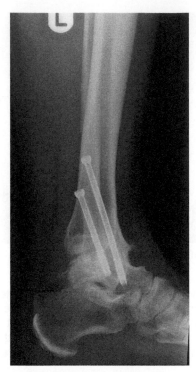

Fig. 10. Radiograph 12 weeks postoperatively, lateral view.

that there is a deep infection, removal of metalwork, drilling out of the screw tracts, and external fixation to maintain the position and then 6 weeks of appropriate antibiotics is recommended.

Prominent screwheads are treated with removal of screws once the fusion is healed.

Nonunion can be treated with rearthroscopic fusion in the first instance. Care should be taken to remove risk factors such as smoking or poor nutritional status. For some cases, open revision with bone grafting might be needed.

Malalignment, such as equinus, should be avoided. Malaligned ankle fusions can be managed with orthotics, revision surgery, osteotomies, and in some cases, a late conversion to total ankle replacement.

Adjacent joint arthrosis is a well-known complication to ankle fusions. Limited evidence shows that arthroscopic fusion represents a lower level of risk and that many patients have preexisting arthritis.[1,2]

POSTOPERATIVE CARE

On the operating table, sterile wound dressings and a below-knee splint is applied.

Before discharge, this can be changed to a below-knee cast.

Although different postoperative regimes have been published, the regime used routinely in the unit has been proved to be reliable. This has not changed for over 10 years.[6,7]

The patient is kept non–weight bearing for the first 2 weeks.

From week 2 to 8 postoperatively, the patient is allowed partial weight bearing in plaster. From postoperative week 8 to 12, full weight bearing in a removable boot is allowed.

Table 1
Summary of outcomes

AAA	Type of Study	Number of Patients/Fusions	Union Rate (%)	Mean Time to Union (wk)	Mean Hospital Stay (d)	Mean Follow-Up (mo)	Other Outcomes/Comments	P Values AAA vs OAA
Abicht & Roukis,[8] 2013	Systematic review[1]	244	91	8	Not stated	24	[1]Including 7 original articles	
Dannawi et al,[5] 2011	Case series	55	91	10	Not stated	63		
Gougoulias et al,[8] 2007	Case series	78	97	12	3.7 ± 4.1	21		
Winson et al,[6] 2005	Case series	105	92	12	4 (1–21)	65	Union rate 95% excluding first 8 cases	
Comparisons AAA vs OAA								
Townshend et al,[2] 2013; AAA	Case series	30	97	Not stated	2.5 ± 1.3[2]	24	Mean AOS score 1 y 17.5[3], 2 y 17.2[4]	[2]P = .05
Townshend et al,[2] 2013; OAA	Case series	27	96	Not stated	3.7 ± 1.8[2]	24	Mean AOS score 1 y 33.5[3], 2 y 29.2[4]	[3]P = .01, [4]P = .05
Nielsen et al,[9] 2008; AAA	Case series	58	95	90% <12[5]	6.6 (3–18)[6]	>12		[5]P<.01
Nielsen et al,[9] 2008; OAA	Case series	48	83	57% <12[5]	8.9 (4–27)[6]	>12		[6]P<.01
O'Brien et al,[10] 1999; AAA	Case series	19	84	Not stated	1.6 (1–4)[7]	Not stated		[7]P<.05
O'Brien et al,[10] 1999; OAA	Case series	17	82	Not stated	3.4 (1–6)[7]	Not stated		
Myerson & Quill,[11] 1990; AAA	Case series	17	94	9[8]	1.5 (1–4)	23		[8]P<.004
Myerson & Quill,[11] 1990; OAA	Case series	16	100	15[8]	4 (2–9)	23		

Hospital stay in days given as mean ± standard deviation or mean (range).
Abbreviations: AOS score, Ankle Osteoarthritis Scale score; OAA, open ankle arthrodesis.

At 12 weeks if clinical and radiological control is judged satisfactory, full weight bearing without protection is allowed **Figs. 9** and **10**.

OUTCOMES

A review of the literature with outcomes is presented in **Table 1**.[2,5–11]

SUMMARY

Arthroscopic ankle arthrodesis is a good/better option for most patients suitable for ankle fusion.

The technique involves careful preparation of joint surfaces and rigid fixation.

Results are similar to those of open ankle arthrodesis, with lower complication rates.

SUPPLEMENTARY DATA

Supplementary data related to this article can be found online at http://dx.doi.org/10.1016/j.fcl.2014.10.008.

REFERENCES

1. Daniels TR, Younger AS, Penner M, et al. Intermediate-term results of total ankle replacement and ankle arthrodesis: a COFAS multicenter study. J Bone Joint Surg Am 2014;96(2):135–42.
2. Townshend D, Di Silvestro M, Krause F, et al. Arthroscopic versus open ankle arthrodesis: a multicenter comparative case series. J Bone Joint Surg Am 2013; 95(2):98–102.
3. Pakzad H, Thevendran G, Penner MJ, et al. Factors associated with longer length of hospital stay after primary elective ankle surgery for end-stage ankle arthritis. J Bone Joint Surg Am 2014;96(1):32–9.
4. Peterson KS, Lee MS, Buddecke DE. Arthroscopic versus open ankle arthrodesis: a retrospective cost analysis. J Foot Ankle Surg 2010;49(3):242–7.
5. Dannawi Z, Nawabi DH, Patel A, et al. Arthroscopic ankle arthrodesis: are results reproducible irrespective of pre-operative deformity? Foot Ankle Surg 2011;17(4): 294–9.
6. Winson IG, Robinson DE, Allen PE. Arthroscopic ankle arthrodesis. J Bone Joint Surg Br 2005;87(3):343–7.
7. Gougoulias NE, Agathangelidis FG, Parsons SW. Arthroscopic ankle arthrodesis. Foot Ankle Int 2007;28(6):695–706.
8. Abicht BP, Roukis TS. Incidence of nonunion after isolated arthroscopic ankle arthrodesis. Arthroscopy 2013;29(5):949–54.
9. Nielsen KK, Linde F, Jensen NC. The outcome of arthroscopic and open surgery ankle arthrodesis: a comparative retrospective study on 107 patients. Foot Ankle Surg 2008;14(3):153–7.
10. O'Brien TS, Hart TS, Shereff MJ, et al. Open versus arthroscopic ankle arthrodesis: a comparative study. Foot Ankle Int 1999;20(6):368–74.
11. Myerson MS, Quill G. Ankle arthrodesis. A comparison of an arthroscopic and an open method of treatment. Clin Orthop Relat Res 1991;268:84–95.

Endoscopic Coalition Resection

Davide Edoardo Bonasia, MD[a],*, Phinit Phisitkul, MD[b], Annunziato Amendola, MD[b]

KEYWORDS

- Tarsal coalition • Arthroscopy • Endoscopy • Foot • Talocalcaneal
- Calcaneonavicular

KEY POINTS

- Indications and contraindications have been described for endoscopic resection of calcaneonavicular coalitions (CNC) and talocalcaneal coalitions (TCC) coalitions.
- Preoperative planning has been described for CNC and TCC.
- Surgical technique has been described for CNC resection, including, patient's preparation, portal placement, and surgical steps.
- Surgical technique has been described for TCC resection, including patient preparation, portal placement, and surgical steps.
- The results for open and endoscopic CNC and TCC resection have been described.

INTRODUCTION

Tarsal coalition occurs in 1% to 6% of the population[1–3] and can be bilateral in approximately 50% to 60% of the cases.[1] Talocalcaneal coalitions (TCC) and calcaneonavicular coalitions (CNC) account, respectively, for approximately 53% and 37% of all tarsal coalitions.[4] According to the predominant tissue, tarsal coalitions are divided into synostosis (bone), synchondrosis (cartilage), and syndesmosis (fibrous tissue).

Asymptomatic coalitions do not need treatment, whereas the management of painful coalitions still remains controversial. At present, the standard first-line approach is the conservative treatment.[1,3] If conservative management fails, surgical treatment may be indicated. Different open techniques have been described and still represent the gold standard for TCC and CNC excision, with or without interposition

---

The authors have nothing to disclose regarding this article.

[a] Department of Orthopaedics and Traumatology, AO Città della Salute e della Scienza – Presidio CTO, University of Torino, Via Zuretti 29, Torino 10100, Italy; [b] Department of Orthopaedics and Rehabilitation, University of Iowa Hospitals and Clinics, University of Iowa, 200 Hawkins Drive, Iowa City, IA 52242, USA
* Corresponding author. Via Lamarmora 26, Torino 10128, Italy.
E-mail address: davidebonasia@virgilio.it

Foot Ankle Clin N Am 20 (2015) 81–91
http://dx.doi.org/10.1016/j.fcl.2014.10.006
1083-7515/15/$ – see front matter © 2015 Elsevier Inc. All rights reserved.

foot.theclinics.com

material (bone wax, fat, muscle, and tendon grafts).[1,3] Endoscopic/arthroscopic resection of coalitions have been described for CNC[5–8] and TCC,[3] with the goals of achieving an adequate resection with less perioperative morbidity and faster recovery. Although endoscopic/arthroscopic surgery of the foot and ankle has significantly evolved in the past decades and has been proved to be safe, endoscopic resection of tarsal coalition still remains an experimental procedure with only few case reports in the literature. The goal of this article is to review indications, surgical technique, complications, and results of endoscopic/arthroscopic resection of tarsal coalition.

INDICATIONS/CONTRAINDICATIONS

Initially, conservative treatment is attempted for symptomatic coalitions. In mildly symptomatic cases, this includes: (1) activity modifications, (2) medial arch supports, (3) University of California Biomechanics Laboratory orthoses, (4) nonsteroidal antiinflammatory drugs, and (5) physical therapy.[1,3] In cases of severe pain or persistent symptoms despite conservative management, a 4- to 6-week cast immobilization is recommended.[1,3] Greater success rate of conservative therapy is achieved in patients with TCCs. CNCs are less likely to respond to conservative treatment.[9]

If conservative management fails, surgical treatment is considered. Open resection, subtalar arthrodesis, and triple arthrodesis have been described. Triple arthrodesis is widely accepted in case of severe degenerative changes in the tarsal joints, which represent a contraindication to resection or isolated subtalar arthrodesis.[1,3] Considering the young age at presentation, when the tarsal joints are preserved, open resection should be considered.[1,3] Tarsal coalition resection can be performed by either arthroscopic or open techniques. **Tables 1** and **2** summarize the main indications/contraindications for arthroscopic CNC and TCC coalition resection.

SURGICAL TECHNIQUE/PROCEDURE
Preoperative Planning

Plain radiographs should include weight-bearing dorsal plantar, and lateral views as well as a non–weight-bearing 45° oblique view of both feet. The posterior hindfoot alignment view may be useful to assess the malalignment in the planovalgus and cavovarus foot.[10] The Harris-Beath view, or ski jump view, has been used to identify talocalcaneal synostosis.[11] The axial view of the subtalar joint is usually difficult to obtain.[12,13] The "C" sign, talar beaking at the talonavicular joint, dysmorphic sustentaculum tali, loss of the normal middle facet, and shortening of the talar neck are

Table 1	
Indication for endoscopic calcaneonavicular resection	
Indications	**Contraindications**
Persistent pain, despite conservative treatment	Asymptomatic patients with no ROM limitations
Significant limitation of ankle and subtalar joints ROM	Active infection Revision surgery
	Significant and symptomatic tarsal joint changes

Abbreviation: ROM, range of motion.

Table 2
Indication for arthroscopic talocalcaneal resection

Indications	Contraindications
Persistent pain, despite conservative treatment	Asymptomatic patients
Posterior facet coalition	Anterior or middle facet coalition
Nonarthritic subtalar and tarsal joints	Arthritic subtalar and/or tarsal joints
<50% of subtalar joint involved	>50% of subtalar joint involved
	Revision surgery
	Previous open surgery around arthroscopic portals
	Active infection
	Absence of posterior tibial pulses

typical radiological findings.[1] Computed tomography is the gold standard imaging technique in assessing the size and location of the coalition, whereas and magnetic resonance imaging is more useful in identifying the histologic pattern of the coalition, mostly when it is nonosseous (**Figs. 1** and **2**).[1]

CNC Endoscopic Resection

Preparation and patient positioning

- *Anesthesia*: General with a regional block or spinal
- *Preoperative antibiotic prophylaxis*: Cefazolin, 2 g, intravenously (IV) for adults and 30 mg/kg for children.[14]
- *Patient's position*: Supine with a bump under the ipsilateral hip and a tourniquet at the proximal thigh.

Portal placement and instrumentation

- *Visualization portal.* The superficial peroneal nerve is located subcutaneously with inversion of the foot and flexion of the toes. The primary visualization portal is established slightly dorsal to the Gissane angle. The skin incision is made, and then blunt dissection is performed with a mosquito clamp until bone contact (**Fig. 3**).[5]
- *Working portal.* The working portal is established with a needle under fluoroscopic control and is located directly over the CNC coalition in the space

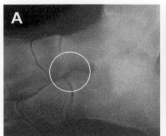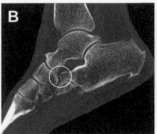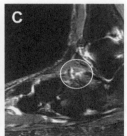

Fig. 1. Fibrous CNC coalition (*white circle*) in (*A*) oblique foot view, (*B*) sagittal computed tomographic scan, and (*C*) sagittal magnetic resonance imaging.

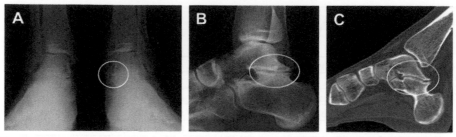

Fig. 2. Posteromedial TCC fibrous coalition of the left foot. (*A*) Anteroposterior views of both ankle, (*B*) lateral view of the left ankle, and (*C*) axial computed tomographic scan of the foot and ankle showing unilateral left foot fibrous coalition (*white circle*).

between the talonavicular and calcaneocuboid joints.[5] The working portal is generally located less than 1 cm dorsal and medial to the superficial peroneal nerve. After skin incision, the mosquito clamp is used for blunt dissection and opened in front of the arthroscope to improve visualization (see **Fig. 3**).

- *Accessory visualization portal.* If the deep part of the anteromedial calcaneal process is not well visualized, an accessory visualization portal can be established under image intensifier at the medial side of the extensor hallucis tendon at the level of the talonavicular joint.[5]
- *Alternative portal placement.* Alternatively, the visualization portal can be placed 0.5 cm anterior to the anterolateral corner of the calcaneus and the working portal at the medial border of the extensor tendons (2 cm medial to the visualization portal) (**Fig. 4**).[8]
- *Instrumentation*: 2.7- or 4.0-mm 30° arthroscope and 2.7- or 4.0-mm shaver and burr.

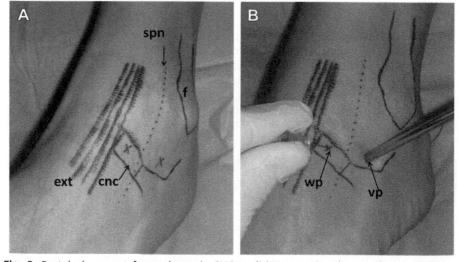

Fig. 3. Portal placement for endoscopic CNC coalition resection (see text). (*A*) Anatomic landmarks with respect to the portals (marked with an X on the patient's skin). ext, Extensor tendons; f, fibula; spn, superficial peroneal nerve. (*B*) Placement for the visualization portal (vp) and working portal (wp). The wp is established with a needle under fluoroscopic and arthroscopic control.

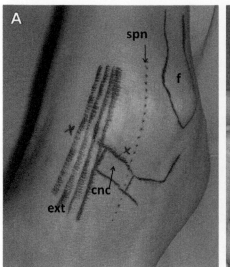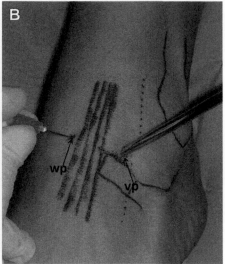

Fig. 4. Alternative portal placement (portals marked with an X on the patient's skin). (*A*) Anatomic landmarks with respect to the portals (marked with an X on the patient's skin). ext, Extensor tendons; f, fibula; spn, superficial peroneal nerve. (*B*) Note how the visualization portal (vp) is more medial compared with that in **Fig. 2** and the working portal (wp) is medial to the extensor tendons (see text).

Surgical procedure

- Step 1 (*visualization*): The soft tissue around the CNC coalition is debrided with an arthroscopic shaver through the working portal.
- Step 2 (*coalition resection*): The CNC coalition is resected with an arthroscopic burr through the working portal. The bone bar is resected until the medial side of the calcaneocuboid joint, the lateral side of the taloclavicular joint, and the plantar lateral aspect of the talar head are clearly seen.[5] The deep part of the anteromedial process can be fully visualized through the accessory visualization portal, in order to ensure adequate bone resection. Inversion and eversion maneuvers are performed to confirm the mobility between the navicular bone and the calcaneus and to exclude impingement between calcaneus and navicular bone.
- Step 3 (*intraoperative fluoroscopy*): The adequacy of bone resection is confirmed with intraoperative oblique views of the foot. Generally, 1 cm separation between the anteromedial process of the calcaneus and the navicular bone is required (**Fig. 5**).

TCC Arthroscopic Resection

Preparation and patient positioning

- *Anesthesia*: General with a regional block or spinal
- *Preoperative antibiotic prophylaxis*: Cefazolin, 2 g, IV for adults and 30 mg/kg for children.[14]
- *Patient's position*: Prone with the feet hanging off the operative table and adequate padding under head, chest, knees, elbows, and shins. Tourniquet is positioned at the proximal thigh

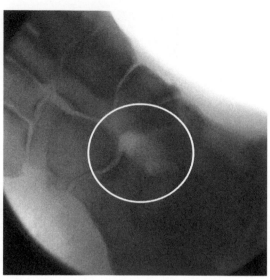

Fig. 5. Fluoroscopy after CNC resection (same case of **Fig. 1**). Note that at least 1-cm resection has been achieved and considered adequate (*white circle*).

Portal placement and instrumentation

- *Posterolateral (PL) portal*: The Achilles tendon and the medial and lateral malleoli are marked with a surgical pen. With the ankle in the neutral position, a line is drawn from the tip of the lateral malleolus to the Achilles tendon, parallel to the foot sole. The PL portal is placed above this line, tangential to the Achilles tendon, and made first. An 18-gauge needle is used to inject up to 10 mL of saline into the subtalar joint. Inversion of the foot indicates successful joint instillation. A longitudinal skin incision is made, and a blunt instrument is inserted toward the lateral aspect of the subtalar joint. The arthroscope is then inserted into the lateral recess of the subtalar joint, and the flexor hallucis longus (FHL) is visualized, as the arthroscope is moved medially. The FHL tendon is an important landmark and should always be kept in view medially, in order to avoid damage to the neurovascular bundle during the procedure. Passive motion of the great toe assists in the identification of the FHL tendon (**Fig. 6**).[3]
- *Posteromedial (PM) portal*: The PM portal is at the same level as the PL portal, medial and tangential to the Achilles tendon. An 18-gauge needle is inserted into the joint at the level of the PM portal. The needle is visualized with the arthroscope to ensure that it is lateral to the FHL. The PM portal longitudinal skin incision is then made. A mosquito clamp is bluntly introduced into the lateral aspect of the subtalar joint and directed toward the arthroscope. The clamp is used to spread the soft tissue in front of the tip of the lens (see **Fig. 6**).[3]
- *Instrumentation*: 2.7-mm 30° arthroscope and 2.7- or 4.0-mm shaver and burr.

Surgical procedure

- Step 1 (*synovectomy and joint balance*): Synovectomy of the subtalar and ankle joint is carried out with a 4-mm shaver until the coalition is clearly visualized (**Fig. 7**A). The arthroscope is gently passed above the posterior talofibular ligament and below the posterior inferior tibiofibular ligament, in order to enter the ankle joint and perform an arthroscopic evaluation to rule out concomitant ankle pathologies.[3]

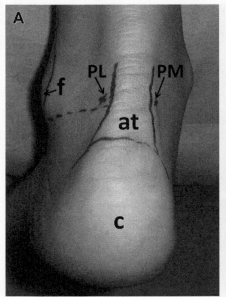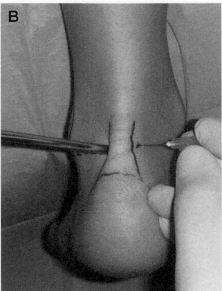

Fig. 6. Portal placement for arthroscopic TCC coalition (see text). (*A*) PL and posteromedial (PM) portals with respect to the anatomic landmarks. at, Achilles tendon; c, calcaneus; f, fibula. (*B*) The PL portal is established first, and the PM portal is performed with a needle after arthroscopic visualization.

- Step 2 (*coalition resection*): Most of the procedure is performed with the arthroscope in the PL and the instruments in the PM portal. In case of nonosseous coalitions, a probe can be inserted between the talus and calcaneus. Gentle levering of the probe can be used to evaluate the subtalar joint motion. In some cases with osseous coalitions, the subtalar joint cannot be visualized. In these cases, the posterior talofibular ligament (PTFL) is used as a landmark: the subtalar joint is located approximately 5 mm below the talar insertion of the PTFL. An acromioplasty burr and a shaver are then used to excise the coalition posteriorly, until healthy cartilage is visualized (see **Fig. 7**B). The excision is extended laterally and medially, according to the size and location of the coalition. On the medial side, the FHL tendon should be always kept medial to the instruments. In order to safely perform the resection anteromedially, the PM corner of the subtalar joint is removed, so that some space (5–7 mm) is created between the FHL and the medial aspect of the subtalar joint. Then, the burr can be advanced anteromedially with an inclination of approximately 30° to the sagittal plane, from posterior/medial to anterior/lateral. In this way, both the FHL and the neurovascular bundle can be preserved.[3]
- Step 3 (*final evaluation*): When healthy cartilage is visualized posteriorly, medially and laterally, and a good subtalar motion is achieved, the resection can be considered complete. A probe can be inserted between talus and calcaneus, and a gentle levering is performed to verify the opening of the joint (see **Fig. 7**C, D). Residual cartilage prominences and bony spurs are finally removed with the shaver or the burr, in order to obtain a smooth surface and avoid irritation to the FHL or posterior ankle impingement. Intraoperative fluoroscopy can also be performed to ensure adequate resection (**Fig. 8**).[3]

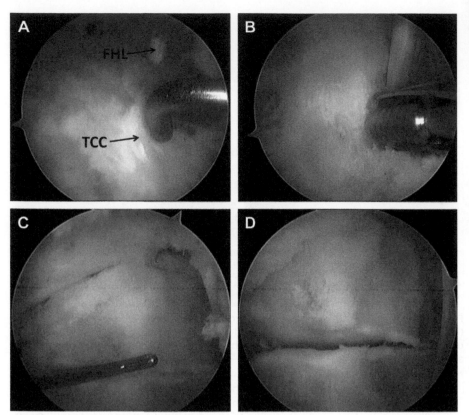

Fig. 7. Arthroscopic resection of the TCC coalition showed in **Fig. 2**. (*A*) The FHL is identified and kept medial with respect to the instruments, in order to avoid neurovascular damages. The TCC coalition is identified and probed. (*B*) Resection is performed with an acromioplasty burr. (*C*) After resection is completed, a probe is used to check subtalar motion. (*D*) Complete motion of the subtalar joint was achieved.

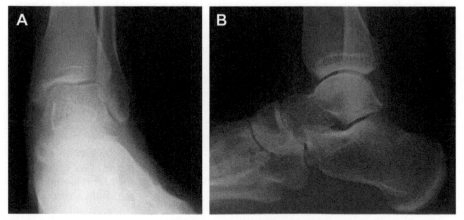

Fig. 8. Postoperative anteroposterior (*A*) and lateral (*B*) views of the ankle (same case shown in **Figs. 2** and **7**).

POSTOPERATIVE CARE

- The patient is discharged the same day, with range of motion exercises and weight bearing as tolerated, in a postoperative boot for pain control.
- Active motion exercises and passive stretching of the first metatarsophalangeal joint are recommended for TCC coalition.

Table 3
Results for open and endoscopic calcaneonavicular and talocalcaneal resection

Author	No. of Cases	Technique	Follow-up	Results
Mitchell & Gibson,[16] 1967	41 CNC	Open excision of bar	6 y	Complete relief of symptoms in 68%
Swiontkowski et al,[17] 1983	39 CNC	Open excision and fat/muscle interposition	4.6 y	Relief of symptoms was complete in 29 cases, almost complete in 7 cases. 90% subtalar motion was restored in 90% of the cases
Gonzalez & Kumar,[18] 1990	75 CNC	Open resection and interposition of the extensor digitorum brevis muscle	2–23 y	Excellent/good (58), fair (3), poor (5)
Mubarak et al,[19] 2009	96 CNC	Open excision and fat interposition	29 mo	87% of the patients returned to sport, whereas 5% showed relapsed and required revision. 74% showed improved subtalar motion and 82% showed improved plantarflexion
Takakura et al,[20] 1991	67 TCC	31 conservative, 33 open excision, 3 open fusion	5.3 y	Results for excision: excellent (24), good (7), fair (2)
Salomao et al,[21] 1992	32 TCC	Open resection and fat interposition		78.1% painless, 21.8% relief of pain
Comfort & Johnson,[22] 1998	20 TCC	Open resection and interposition	29 mo	Good/excellent 77%
Bauer et al,[6] 2010	1 CNC	Endoscopic resection	2 y	American Orthopaedic Foot & Ankle Society (AOFAS) ankle–hindfoot score went from 23 preoperatively to 82 after surgery
Knörr et al,[7] 2011	3 CNC	Endoscopic resection	1 y	Mean AOFAS score rose from 58 preoperatively to 91 at last follow-up
Bernardino et al,[8] 2009	1 CNC	Endoscopic resection	2 y	AOFAS ankle–hindfoot score went from 55 preoperatively to 100 at last follow-up

Data from Refs.[6–8,16–22]

- At 3 weeks from surgery, the boot can be dismissed and the patient advanced to full daily activities.
- At 6 weeks, the patient can be progressed to sports without restrictions.

COMPLICATIONS

No complications have been described for endoscopic CNC resection, because only case reports and small case series have been published. However, theoretic complications include:

- Recurrence of the symptoms
- Inadequate coalition resection
- Injuries to the dorsalis pedis artery and the superficial peroneal nerve
- Injuries to the extensors and peroneus tertius tendons
- Infection and deep venous thrombosis

Although no complications have been specifically described for arthroscopic TCC resection, in 2012 Nickisch and colleagues[15] reported the complications of posterior ankle and hindfoot arthroscopy. Out of 189 ankles, complications were noted in 16 cases (8.5%): 4 patients had plantar numbness, 3 had sural nerve dysesthesia, 4 had Achilles tendon tightness, 2 had complex regional pain syndrome, 2 had an infection, and 1 had a cyst at the PM portal. One case each of plantar numbness and sural nerve dysesthesia failed to resolve. Other theoretic complications after arthroscopic TCC resection include:

- Recurrence of the symptoms
- Inadequate coalition resection
- Injuries to the posterior tibialis artery and the tibial nerve
- Injury to the flexor hallucis longus
- Deep venous thrombosis

OUTCOMES

Relevant results for open and endoscopic resection of CNC and TCC have been summarized in **Table 3**. As shown in **Table 3**, although open resection is a widely used technique for both CNC and TCC, with or without graft interposition, endoscopic resection can still be considered experimental and only few case reports or small case series have been published. However, the endoscopic techniques seem to be safe and produce good results,[8,15] with less local morbidity.

Possible disadvantages of the arthroscopic techniques may be related to: (1) longer learning curve, (2) increased duration of the procedure, (3) damage to neurovascular bundles, and (4) difficulties in using interposition material (ie, bone wax, fat, and split tendons). However, the use of interposition material was not shown to be superior to isolated resection or to reduce recurrence rates.[23–25]

SUMMARY

Although arthroscopic/endoscopic tarsal coalition resection seem to be promising with the possible advantages of faster recovery and reduced local morbidity, this techniques has a long learning curve. Larger case series are needed to definitely confirm the reliability of the arthroscopic/endoscopic procedures and allow a comparison with traditional open techniques.

REFERENCES

1. Lemley F, Berlet G, Hill K, et al. Current concepts review: tarsal coalition. Foot Ankle Int 2006;27:1163–9.
2. Wray JB, Herndon CN. Hereditary transmission of congenital coalition of the calcaneus to the navicular. J Bone Joint Surg Am 1963;45:365–72.
3. Bonasia DE, Phisitkul P, Saltzman CL, et al. Arthroscopic resection of talocalcaneal coalitions. Arthroscopy 2011;27:430–5.
4. Stormont DM, Peterson HA. The relative incidence of tarsal coalition. Clin Orthop Relat Res 1983;(181):28–36.
5. Lui TH. Arthroscopic resection of the calcaneonavicular coalition or the "too long" anterior process of the calcaneus. Arthroscopy 2006;22:903.e1–4.
6. Bauer T, Golano P, Hardy P. Endoscopic resection of a calcaneonavicular coalition. Knee Surg Sports Traumatol Arthrosc 2010;18:669–72.
7. Knörr J, Accadbled F, Abid A, et al. Arthroscopic treatment of calcaneonavicular coalition in children. Orthop Traumatol Surg Res 2011;97:565–8.
8. Bernardino CM, Golanó P, Garcia MA, et al. Experimental model in cadavera of arthroscopic resection of calcaneonavicular coalition and its first in-vivo application: preliminary communication. J Pediatr Orthop B 2009;18:347–53.
9. Bohne WH. Tarsal coalition. Curr Opin Pediatr 2001;13:29–35.
10. Saltzman CL, el-Khoury GY. The hindfoot alignment view. Foot Ankle Int 1995;16: 572–6.
11. Harris RI, Beath T. Etiology of peroneal spastic flat foot. J Bone Joint Surg Br 1948;30:624–34.
12. Cowell HR. Talocalcaneal coalition and new causes of peroneal spastic flatfoot. Clin Orthop Relat Res 1972;85:16–22.
13. Jayakumar S, Cowell HR. Rigid flatfoot. Clin Orthop Relat Res 1977;(122):77–84.
14. Bratzler DW, Dellinger EP, Olsen KM, et al. Clinical practice guidelines for antimicrobial prophylaxis in surgery. Am J Health Syst Pharm 2013;1(70):195–283.
15. Nickisch F, Barg A, Saltzman CL, et al. Postoperative complications of posterior ankle and hindfoot arthroscopy. J Bone Joint Surg Am 2012;94:439–46.
16. Mitchell GP, Gibson JM. Excision of calcaneo-navicular bar for painful spasmodic flat foot. J Bone Joint Surg Br 1967;49:281–7.
17. Swiontkowski MF, Scranton PE, Hansen S. Tarsal coalitions: long-term results of surgical treatment. J Pediatr Orthop 1983;3:287–92.
18. Gonzalez P, Kumar SJ. Calcaneonavicular coalition treated by resection and interposition of the extensor digitorum brevis muscle. J Bone Joint Surg Am 1990;72:71–7.
19. Mubarak SJ, Patel PN, Upasani VV, et al. Calcaneonavicular coalition: treatment by excision and fat graft. J Pediatr Orthop 2009;29:418–26.
20. Takakura Y, Sugimoto K, Tanaka Y, et al. Symptomatic talocalcaneal coalition: its clinical significance and treatment. Clin Orthop Relat Res 1991;(269):249–56.
21. Salomao O, Napoli MM, de Carvalho Junior AE, et al. Talocalcaneal coalition: diagnosis and surgical management. Foot Ankle 1992;13:251–6.
22. Comfort TK, Johnson LO. Resection for symptomatic talocalcaneal coalition. J Pediatr Orthop 1998;18:283–8.
23. Kitaoka HB, Wikenheiser MA, Shaughnessy WJ, et al. Gait abnormalities following resection of talocalcaneal coalition. J Bone Joint Surg Am 1997;79:369–74.
24. McCormack TJ, Olney B, Asher M. Talocalcaneal coalition resection: a 10-year follow-up. J Pediatr Orthop 1997;17:13–5.
25. Kumar SJ, Guille JT, Lee MS, et al. Osseous and non-osseous coalition of the middle facet of the talocalcaneal joint. J Bone Joint Surg Am 1992;74:529–35.

Subtalar Arthroscopy

Indications, Technique and Results

Gerardo Muñoz, MD, PhD*, Sergio Eckholt, MD

KEYWORDS

- Hindfoot • Subtalar joint • Sinus tarsi syndrome • Posttraumatic ankle pain
- Subtalar osteochondral lesion • Os trigonum • Subtalar synovitis
- Subtalar arthroscopy

KEY POINTS

- Because of its complex anatomy, subtalar pathologic conditions are a challenge to diagnose and treat.
- Surgical management is considered after an appropriate trial of conservative treatment has failed.
- Subtalar arthroscopy has evolved as an important tool in the study and treatment of numerous subtalar pathologic conditions, particularly sinus tarsi syndrome.
- Although results have been encouraging, further technique and instrument development and long-term studies are needed to improve and validate subtalar arthroscopy.

INTRODUCTION: NATURE OF THE PROBLEM

Traditional open hindfoot surgery can have a relatively high complication rate because of the special soft tissue characteristics that surround the subtalar joint. Currently, small joint arthroscopic procedures including the subtalar joint have evolved and expanded in its indications, thereby reducing complications attributed to open surgical techniques. Improved techniques, increased surgeon experience, and the development of specialized small joint instrumentation have permitted minimally invasive subtalar surgery to address many hindfoot pathologic conditions.

One of the initial challenges with subtalar arthroscopic techniques is the anatomic disposition of the articular facets, especially the posterior joint that runs semi–concave-convex in 2 planes. This joint provides a narrow space in which to work. These issues require a long learning curve for the surgeon to acquire the necessary skills to safely and effectively operate in this zone.

The authors have nothing to disclose.
Departamento de Ortopedia y Traumatologia, Clinica Las Condes, Lo Fontecilla 441, Las Condes, Santiago 7591046, Chile
* Corresponding author.
E-mail address: gmunoz@clc.cl

Foot Ankle Clin N Am 20 (2015) 93–108
http://dx.doi.org/10.1016/j.fcl.2014.10.010
foot.theclinics.com

Although a relatively small number of reports on subtalar arthroscopy exists in the literature, they have described their arthroscopic findings, confirmed a similar range of pathologic conditions that affect other joints, and developed procedures to address these conditions. They also identified separate clinical identities to treat. For example, sinus tarsi syndrome was considered a vague preoperative diagnosis that corresponded to different entities, for which available imaging tools were not able to delineate its origin.

For other known pathologic conditions, such as subtalar arthrosis, osteochondral lesions, chronic synovitis, chondromalacia, arthrofibrosis, osteophytes, loose bodies, os trigonum syndrome, and others, imaging modalities including MRI, computed tomography (CT), and single-photon emission CT (SPECT-CT) have better accuracy in diagnosis. Anesthetic injections continue to play a predominant role in differentiating pain between the ankle and subtalar joint and surrounding soft tissues.

INDICATIONS/CONTRAINDICATIONS

Subtalar arthroscopy is used as a diagnostic and therapeutic tool for intra- or extra-articular pathologic conditions when they are resistant to conservative treatment. Indications include a persistent subtalar pain, subtalar impingement, chronic synovitis, debridement and treatment of cartilage defects and cystic lesions, removal of osteophytes, release of adhesion in arthrofibrosis, removal of loose bodies, evaluation and reduction of hindfoot fractures, arthroscopic arthrodesis of subtalar joint, and removal of posterior facet talocalcaneal coalition (**Box 1**).[1,2]

With sinus tarsi syndrome, a more accurate diagnosis can be made with this procedure, improving the treatment plan. Ahn and coworkers[3] operated on 31 patients with a preoperative diagnosis of sinus tarsi syndrome that changed at the time of arthroscopy. The postoperative diagnoses included interosseous ligament tears (32%), mild degenerative arthritis (16%), intra-articular loose body (16%), osteochondral fractures (23%), and fibrous coalition (13%). In another study with 33 consecutive cases (mean follow-up, 24 months), arthroscopic findings showed partial tear of the interosseous talocalcaneal ligament in 29 cases, synovitis in 18, partial tear of the cervical ligament in 11, arthrofibrosis in 8, and soft-tissue impingement in 7. The mean visual analog scale score improved from 7.3 points preoperatively to 2.7 points postoperatively, and the mean American Orthopaedic Foot and Ankle Society (AOFAS) Ankle-Hindfoot Score improved from 43.1 points preoperatively to 86.2 points postoperatively, with 87% excellent and good results (**Fig. 1**).[4]

Box 1 Indications and procedures	
Indication	**Procedure**
Persistent subtalar pain	Inspection
Soft tissue subtalar impingement (usually scared ligaments)	Tissue removal
Chronic synovitis	Synovectomy
Osteochondral lesion	Debridement, drilling, and microfractures
Symptomatic subtalar coalition	Coalition removal if possible or arthrodesis
Arthrofibrosis	Arthrofibrolysis
Loose bodies	Bodies removal
Control of articular internal fixation	
Degenerative articular disease	Debridement when useful or athrodesis
Os trigonum syndrome	Excision

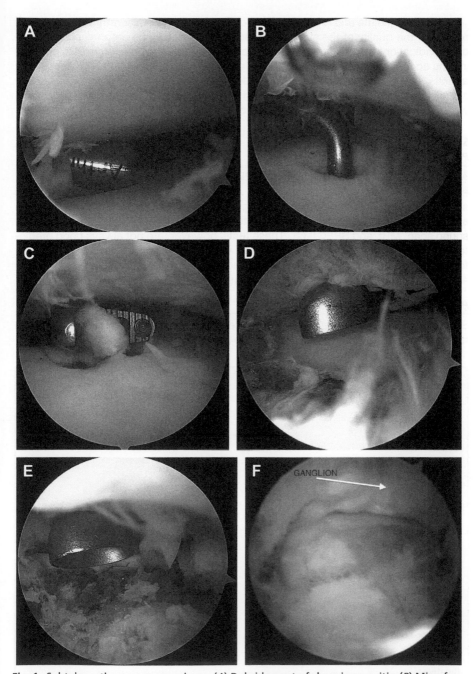

Fig. 1. Subtalar arthroscopy procedures. (*A*) Debridement of chronic synovitis. (*B*) Microfracture of calcaneal subtalar facet. (*C*) Loose body removal. (*D*) Posterior instrumentation. (*E*) Chondral curettage for subtalar arthrodesis. (*F*) Subtalar ganglion from the talocalcaneal ligament in the posterior subtalar joint border producing posterior soft tissue impingement (*arrow*).

There are absolute and relative contraindications for a subtalar arthroscopy directly related to the quality of the surrounding soft tissues and bone deformities. Absolute contraindications include advanced osteoarthritis or severe bone deformities preventing the access to the joint and local soft tissue infection because of the risk of septic arthritis. Among the relative contraindications are poor skin quality or poor vascular status, severe edema, and reflex sympathetic dystrophy. Others contraindications will depend on the particular pathologic condition to be treated (**Box 2**).

SURGICAL TECHNIQUE/PROCEDURE
Preoperative Planning

A complete history and physical examination are essential in assessing subtalar joint and associated extra-articular structures. After a clinical diagnosis is made, imaging should be used to reject or confirm the diagnosis. Several different imaging techniques are available for subtalar joint pathology study, including plain radiographs, CT, ultrasound scan, MRI, and SPECT-CT. These tests, however, are not always good predictors of the articular injury when compared with diagnostic arthroscopy. One study found full agreement in only 10%, partial agreement in 50%, and no agreement in 40% between MRI and arthroscopic findings.[5]

Preparation and Patient Positioning

Subtalar arthroscopy is performed under general or regional anesthesia. A regional nerve block is useful for postoperative pain management. A tourniquet can be used

---

Box 2
Indications and contraindications

Indications

Subtalar impingement

Condral lesions

Arthrofibrosis

Loose bodies

Hindfoot fractures assistance

Subtalar arthrodesis

Talocalcaneal coalition

Sinus tarsi syndrome

Contraindication

Absolute

  Soft tissue infection

  Advance osteoarthritis

  Severe bone deformities

Relative

  Poor skin quality

  Poor vascular status

  Severe edema

  Reflex sympathetic dystrophy

over the proximal thigh to prevent bleeding and improve joint visualization but is rarely needed. Patient position depends on the pathologic condition and the portals to be used. Position can be supine, prone, or lateral with the lateral and prone positions most commonly performed (**Fig. 2**).

The use of distraction facilitates joint visualization[6,7] and depends on the tightness of the joint, the location of condition, and the preference of the surgeon. It can be with noninvasive (manually or with soft tissue devices) or invasive methods if further distraction is necessary. Bone distraction is helpful in a tight posterior subtalar joint by increasing the visualized area and the area available to work.[8,9] Disadvantages of invasive distraction include the potential damage to soft tissues and ligamentous structures, pin breakage, neurovascular injury, infection, and fractures of the talus or calcaneus. One study of 52 patients treated with invasive skeletal traction technique did not show complications related to the method of distraction or problems with nerve dysfunction as a result of wire placement or the high-tension traction.[10]

Transcalcaneal (lateral to medial) 2.0-mm pin traction facilitated with a fracture table traction system can be used to provide slight traction that is enough to obtain a wider working space. Care must be taken to avoid fracture, particularly in osteoporotic bone (**Fig. 3**).

SURGICAL APPROACH
Portals

The subtalar joint can be accessed primarily by 2 different approaches: lateral and posterior. For the lateral approach, the anatomic landmarks for portal placement are the lateral malleolus, the sinus tarsi, and the Achilles tendon. Three arthroscopic portals have been described: anterolateral, middle, and posterolateral. The anterolateral portal is placed 2 cm anterior and 1 cm distal to the tip of the fibula. The middle portal is directly over the sinus tarsi, 1 cm anterior to the tip of the fibula. There are no structures at risk in this portal. The posterolateral portal is placed at the level of the tip of the fibula or 0.5 cm proximal, close to the Achilles tendon to avoid injury to the sural nerve (**Fig. 4**).

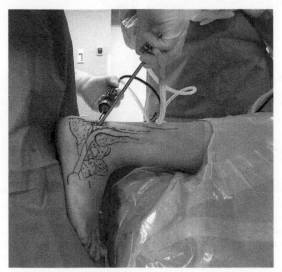

Fig. 2. Patient in prone position with posterior portals. Observe the arthroscope orientation position.

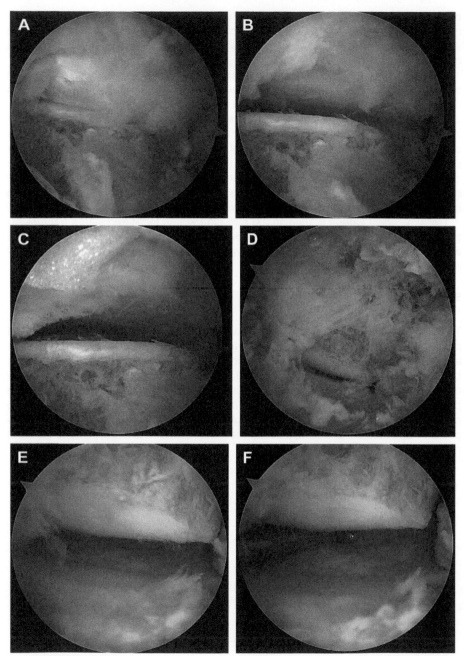

Fig. 3. Role of distraction in subtalar arthroscopy. (*A*) Posterolateral view of subtalar joint without traction. (*B*) Posterolateral view of subtalar joint with mild traction. (*C*) Posterolateral view of subtalar joint with careful full traction. Note the increased space. (*D*) Middle portal view of the middle subtalar joint without traction. (*E*) Middle portal view of the middle subtalar joint with mild traction. (*F*) Middle portal view of the middle subtalar joint with careful full traction.

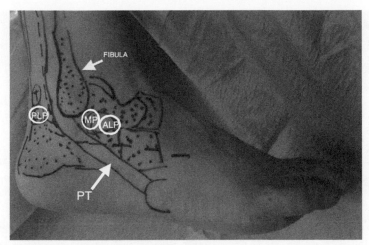

Fig. 4. Landmarks for subtalar portal arthroscopy. ALP, anterolateral portal; MP, middle portal; PLP, posterolateral portal; PT, peroneal tendons.

Two accessory anterolateral and posterolateral portals can be developed as needed for viewing and instrumentation of the joint.[11] The accessory anterolateral portal is a little more anterior and superior to the anterolateral portal and the accessory posterolateral portal is behind the peroneal tendons and lateral to the posterolateral portal, increasing the risk to the sural nerve.

Tryfonidis and coworkers[12] studied the distance between the portals and the sural nerve in a cadaveric study. The median distances of the anterior and middle subtalar portals to the nearest nerve branch (which was either the main sural nerve or one of its branches) was 21.3 mm and 20.9 mm, respectively, and 11.4 mm for the posterior portal. The establishment of the anterior and middle subtalar portals made damage important structures less likely than that of the posterior subtalar portal.

If the surgeon needs to approach the posterior aspect of the subtalar joint, placing the patient prone and assessing the joint with 2 posterior portals is recommended. This occurs in patients with either soft tissue or bony impingement (symptomatic os trigonum). Arthroscopy can be performed using a posterolateral and posteromedial portal.[13] The posterolateral portal is made immediately lateral to the Achilles tendon at the level of or slightly above the tip of the fibula. The posteromedial portal is made just medial to the Achilles tendon at the same level as the posterolateral portal. Sitler and coworkers,[14] in a study of 13 fresh-frozen cadaver specimens, evaluated the relative safety of hindfoot arthroscopy with use of posterolateral and posteromedial portals in the prone position. The average distance to the anatomic structures after dissection was 3.2 mm to the sural nerve, 4.8 mm to the small saphenous vein, 6.4 mm to the tibial nerve, 9.6 mm the posterior tibial artery, 17 mm to the medial calcaneal nerve, and 2.7 mm to the flexor hallucis longus tendon (**Fig. 5**).

There is a medial portal at the medial opening of the tarsal canal. This portal is established by an inside-out technique with a Kirschner wire inserted into the canal under arthroscopic guidance, pointing toward the medial malleolar tip. The portal should exit at the dorsal-distal corner of the medial end of the tarsal canal just behind the sustentaculum tali, above the flexor hallux longus tendon and the medial plantar nerve. It is useful for synovectomy of the medial joint, resection of a talocalcaneal coalition, and assessment and manipulation of a medial calcaneal fracture.[9]

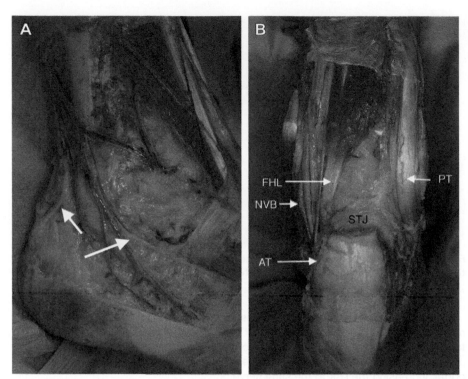

Fig. 5. Anatomic structures to consider. Cadaver dissection (*A*). Arrows show the sural nerve and posterior recurrent branch of sural nerve and its anatomic relations (*B*). AT, Achilles tendon; FHL, flexor hallucis longus tendon; NVB, neurovascular bundle; PT, peroneal tendons; STJ, subtalar joint position.

SURGICAL PROCEDURE

Because of its small size, visualization of the posterior subtalar joint requires the use of small instrumentation. A 2.7-mm 30° short arthroscope is commonly used. Others prefer 10° or 25° similar-diameter arthroscopes. In subtalar joints that are too tight, a 1.9-mm 30° arthroscope is recommended, but there is the potential for instrument breakage. If the objective is to look inside the joint without entering it, it is possible to use a 4.0-mm 30° arthroscope. Siddiqui and colleagues[15] reported good results in 6 patients who underwent subtalar arthroscopy for different disorders. The AOFAS Ankle-Hindfoot Scores improved from 49.6 to 67.3 (range, 53–91) at 3 months and to 75 (range, 54–100) at 6 months. A 2.9-mm 30° lens can offer a wider field of view with minimal increase in diameter. A 2.0- or 2.9-mm shaver set and small joint burr are also needed.

Lateral Approach

By inverting and everting the foot, the sinus tarsi can be palpated in front of the lateral malleolus. Insufflate the joint cavity with 10 mL of normal saline or Ringer's lactate into the sinus tarsi. Remove the needle; the anterolateral portal is made at the same site. Make a small incision with a No. 11 blade and then perform blunt dissection into the joint capsule with a hemostat. The arthroscope is introduced into the subtalar joint in a slightly upward direction, in the orientation of the tarsal canal. For the middle and posterolateral portal, a needle can be used under direct visualization or by palpating the tip of the anteriorly placed arthroscope. Fluoroscopic confirmation of the position of the instruments can be used (**Fig. 6**).

Posterior Approach

In the posterior 2-portal technique, the posterolateral portal is made as described above. After a vertical incision, the subcutaneous layer is bluntly dissected. The arthroscope is directed toward the interdigital webspace between the first and second toe. The level of the posterior subtalar joint can sometimes be distinguished by palpating the prominent posterior talar process. After making the skin incision of the posteromedial portal, a mosquito clamp is introduced and directed toward the arthroscope shaft, which is used as a guide to travel anteriorly in the direction of the posterior subtalar joint. The mosquito clamp is exchanged for the needed instrument to start the procedure.

Systematic examination of the subtalar joint is performed by varying the portal placement of the arthroscope. A 13-point arthroscopic evaluation of the posterior subtalar joint has been advocated by Ferkel[1] and Williams and Ferkel.[16] In the anterolateral portal, the sinus tarsi, interosseous ligament, cervical ligament, and lateral and posterior gutters can be seen. The posterolateral portal enables evaluation of the lateral gutter and lateral compartment, and the middle portal enables visualization of the anterolateral and posteromedial compartments (**Fig. 7**).

COMPLICATIONS AND MANAGEMENT

Complications after subtalar arthroscopy are the same as for any joint arthroscopy: infection, instrument breakage, and damaging the articular cartilage. The main complications specific for this method are injuries of the sural nerve and superficial peroneal nerve at the posterolateral and the anterolateral portal, respectively.

In one study with 33 patients, one case of irritation of the lateral branch of the superficial peroneal nerve at the anterolateral portal was found that was resolved by neurolysis.[4] In another series of 49 cases, 5 minor complications (3 cases of neuritis of the superficial peroneal nerve, 1 patient with sinus tract formation, and 1 superficial wound infection) were reported.[17] In the series by Lee and coworkers[7] of 16 patients who underwent arthroscopic subtalar arthrodesis, only 1 deep infection was found related to screw failure and nonunion in the same patient. Ferkel[1] evaluated 50 patients after posterior subtalar arthroscopy, with an average follow-up of 32 months, and found no major complications (**Table 1**).

POSTOPERATIVE CARE

After the surgery, a compression dressing is applied from midleg to the toes with instructions to keep the foot elevated as often as possible for the first several days to avoid excessive postoperative swelling. Nonsteroidal anti-inflammatory oral medication and icing is recommended to limit swelling and pain. Early range-of-motion exercises of the foot and ankle may be stimulated several times per day immediately after surgery to prevent stiffness of the subtalar joint. Weight bearing as tolerated is recommended from the first postoperative day followed by a gradual progression to full weight bearing,[18] except when severe osseous disease is treated, in which case the indication is modified accordingly. Sutures are removed approximately 7 to 10 days after the procedure.

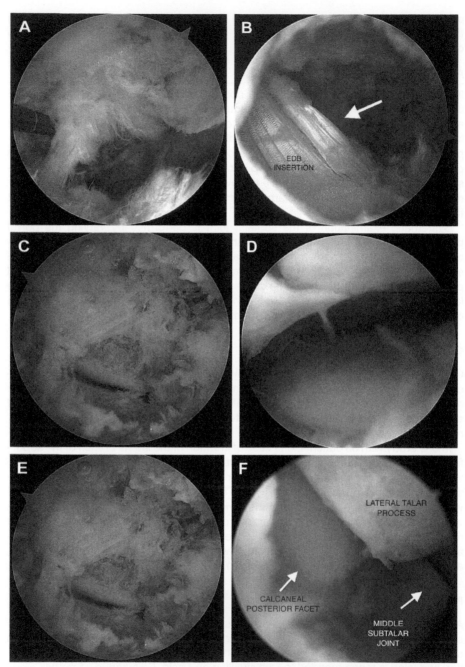

Fig. 6. Observe different views of anterolateral and middle portals. (*A–C*) Anterolateral portal view. (*A*) Partial removal of an interosseous scarred ligament producing impingement. (*B*) Interosseuos ligaments and sinus tarsi insertion of extensor digitorum brevis tendon (EDB). (*C*) Middle subtalar joint. (*D–F*) Middle portal view. (*D*) Posterior subtalar joint. (*E*) Similar view of anterolateral portal of middle joint. (*F*) Arrows show relationship between calcaneal facet, lateral talar process, and middle subtalar joint.

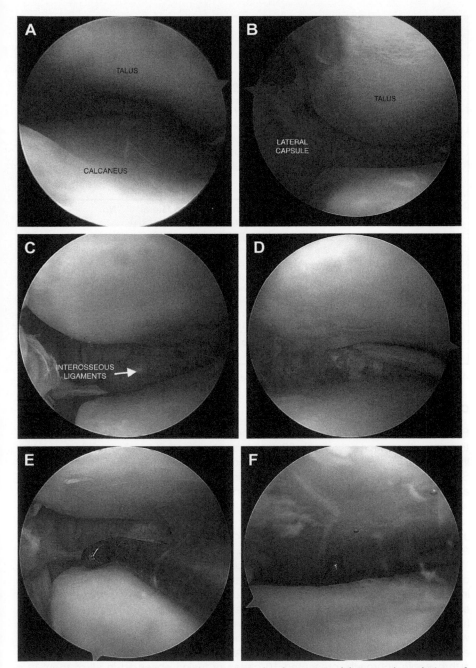

Fig. 7. Posterolateral portal view. (*A*) Intra-articular facet view. (*B*) Posterolateral view of lateral recess and it capsule. (*C*) Intra-articular view of the interosseous ligament in sinus tarsi. (*D*) Posterolateral accessory portal view orientated to the posteromedial joint. (*E*) Posterolateral view palpating chondral defects. (*F*) Posterolateral view and anterolateral instrumentation.

Table 1
Subtalar arthroscopy complications

Author, Year	N	Mean Follow-Up	Complication (%)	Type of Complication	Traction
Frey et al,[17] 1999	49	54 mo	10.2	3 neuritis involving branches of the superficial peroneal nerve, 1 sinus tract formation, and 1 superficial wound infection	No
Oloff et al,[24] 2001	29	18 mo	0	No	Not routinely used
Lee et al,[4] 2008	33	24 mo	3	1 irritation of the lateral branch of the superficial peroneal nerve	No
Ahn et al,[3] 2009	115	42 mo	2.6	1 neuritis involving the branches of the superficial peroneal nerve, 1 superficial wound infection, and 1 hardware removal owing to irritation	No
Beals et al,[10] 2010	14	n/r	0	No	Yes (transcalcaneal)

Abbreviation: n/r, not reported by authors of the mentioned article.

OUTCOMES

Rammelt and coworkers[19] in 59 cases found that despite a seemingly accurate reduction, the arthroscope detected in 22% of cases a step off of 1 to 2 mm, which resulted in a second reduction (**Table 2**). They reported an average AOFAS Ankle-Hindfoot Score of 94 points after 1 year of follow-up in 15 patients treated with arthroscopically assisted percutaneous reduction of intra-articular calcaneus fractures. Sitte and coworkers[20] had good clinical and radiologic results in 2 patients with talar body fractures treated with osteosynthesis using hindfoot and subtalar arthroscopy as auxiliary methods to control the reduction and screw placement, with AOFAS Ankle-Hindfoot Score of 75 and 100 points, respectively, at 6 months.

With arthroscopic subtalar arthrodesis, Lee and colleagues[7] reported a union rate of 94% at a mean of 11 weeks and the mean modified AOFAS Ankle-Hindfoot Score improved from 35 points preoperatively to 84 points at final follow-up. Nonunion occurred in 1 case with no other postoperative complications. Glanzmann and Sanhueza-Hernandez[21] reported a 100% union rate in 41 cases at a mean of 11 weeks with average modified AOFAS Ankle-Hindfoot Score improved from 53 points preoperatively to 84 points at final follow-up. Albert and coworkers,[22] with a posterior arthroscopic approach, presented 10 cases of fusion observed in all of them at a maximum of 9 weeks with mean average AOFAS Ankle-Hindfoot Score improved from 47 to 78. No complications were noted related to the technique at 1 year follow-up.

In a study[23] of 10 patients who underwent subtalar arthroscopy for persistent pain in the subfibular area after open reduction and internal fixation for intra-articular calcaneal fractures, 8 patients (80%) had considerable pain relief and did not require further

Table 2
Subtalar arthroscopy results

Author, Year	N	Mean Follow-Up	Postoperative Diagnosis	AOFAS Score	Other Outcome
Frey et al,[17] 1999	49	54 mo	36 interosseous ligament injury, 7 arthrofibrosis, 4 degenerative joint disease, and 2 fibrous coalition of the calcaneonavicular joint	n/r	47% excellent results, 47% good results, and 6% poor results.
Oloff et al,[24] 2001	29	18 mo	29 synovitis, 1 chondromalacia/degenerative joint disease, 2 arthrofibrosis, 1 os trigonum, 2 interosseous talocalcaneal ligament attenuation/tear, and 1 calcium pyrophosphate disease	85 postoperative	n/r
Lee et al,[4] 2008	33	24 mo	29 partial tear of the interosseous talocalcaneal ligament, 18 synovitis, 11 partial tear of the cervical ligament, 8 arthrofibrosis, and 7 soft tissue impingement	43.1–86.2	VAS 7.3 to 2.7
Ahn et al,[3] 2009	115	42 mo	31 subtalar synovitis, 9 mild degenerative disease, 6 chondromalacia, 11 loose body, 10 arthrofibrosis, 8 symptomatic os trigonum, 6 osteochondral lesion of the talus, 26 severe degenerative joint disease, 10 calcaneal fracture, 2 talar fracture, and 1 calcaneal tumor	33–88 subtalar fusion group 69–89 other-than-fusion group	97% satisfaction
Siddiqui et al,[15] 2010	6	3 and 6 mo	2 posttraumatic subtalar arthrofibrosis, 2 subtalar osteoarthritis, 1 osteochondral lesion, and 1 subtalar gouty arthritis	49.6–67.3 at 3 mo and 75 at 6 mo	n/r

Abbreviations: n/r, not reported by authors of the mentioned article; VAS, visual analog scale.

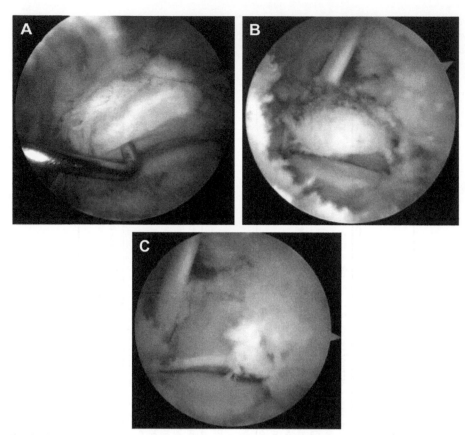

Fig. 8. Os Trigonum removal. (*A*) Os trigonum palpation. (*B*) The relationship between an os trigonum and the flexor hallucis longus tendon. (*C*) View after removal.

local injection or surgical management. The preoperative AOFAS Ankle-Hindfoot Score for the whole group was 69.9 points (range, 68–74 points), which was improved postoperatively to 77.2 points (range, 48–90 points).

In the largest series of cases (115 patients), which included a range of subtalar pathologic conditions, with a mean follow-up period of 42 months, the mean modified AOFAS Ankle-Hindfoot Score in the subtalar fusion group was increased from 33 points preoperatively to 84 points postoperatively, and the mean AOFAS Ankle-Hindfoot Score in the other-than-fusion group increased from 69 points preoperatively to 89 points postoperatively. Ninety-seven percent of patients were satisfied with the procedure, and there were no serious complications.[3] Oloff and co-workers[24] showed similar results in their series of 29 cases, with a mean postoperative AOFAS Ankle-Hindfoot Score of 85 points and a mean return to full activity of 4 months (**Fig. 8**).

SUMMARY

Subtalar pain comprises a wide spectrum of pathologic conditions, mostly secondary to trauma, and the still questioned sinus tarsi syndrome. Conservative treatment is broadly effective in most cases; however, the use of subtalar arthroscopy has expanded when nonoperative management fails or when a more accurate diagnosis is necessary. Although several imaging techniques are available for the workup of subtalar joint pathologic conditions, these techniques are not always as effective as arthroscopy.

The therapeutic results with the use of arthroscopy are encouraging; however, the reports available compare a wide range of pathologic conditions and use different surgical techniques, which means that often the results are not comparable. Nevertheless, arthroscopy is a valuable tool that should be offered to patients with these diagnoses.

REFERENCES

1. Ferkel RD, Small HN, Gittins JE. Complications in foot and ankle arthroscopy. Clin Orthop 2001;391:89–104.
2. Lundeen RO. Arthroscopic fusion of the ankle and subtalar joint. Clin Podiatr Med Surg 1994;11(3):395–406.
3. Ahn JH, Lee SK, Kim KJ, et al. Subtalar arthroscopic procedures for the treatment of subtalar pathologic conditions: 115 consecutive cases. Orthopedics 2009; 32(12):891.
4. Lee KB, Bai LB, Song EK, et al. Subtalar arthroscopy for sinus Tarsi syndrome: arthroscopic findings and clinical outcomes of 33 consecutive cases. Arthroscopy 2008;24(10):1130–4.
5. Lee KB, Bai LB, Park JG, et al. Efficacy of MRI versus arthroscopy for evaluation of sinus tarsi syndrome. Foot Ankle Int 2008;29(11):1111–6.
6. Lee KB, Saltzman CL, Suh JS, et al. A posterior 3-portal arthroscopic approach for isolated subtalar arthrodesis. Arthroscopy 2008;24(11):1306–10.
7. Lee K, Park CH, Seon JK, et al. Arthroscopic subtalar arthrodesis using a posterior 2-portal approach in the prone position. Arthroscopy 2010;26(2):230–8.
8. Kim HN, Ryu SR, Park JM, et al. Subtalar arthroscopy with calcaneal skeletal traction in a hanging position. J Foot Ankle Surg 2012;51(6):816–9.
9. Mekhail AO, Heck BE, Ebraheim NA, et al. Arthroscopy of the subtalar joint: establishing a medial portal. Foot Ankle Int 1995;16(7):427–32.
10. Beals TC, Junko JT, Amendola A, et al. Minimally invasive distraction technique for prone posterior ankle and subtalar arthroscopy. Foot Ankle Int 2010;31(4): 316–9.
11. Frey C, Gasser S, Feder K. Arthroscopy of the subtalar joint. Foot Ankle Int 1994; 15(8):424–8.
12. Tryfonidis M, Whitfield CG, Charalambous CP, et al. The distance between the sural nerve and ideal portal placements in lateral subtalar arthroscopy: a cadaveric study. Foot Ankle Int 2008;29(8):842–4.
13. Van Dijk CN, Scholten PE, Krips R. A 2-portal endoscopic approach for diagnosis and treatment of posterior ankle pathology. Arthroscopy 2000;16(8):871–6.
14. Sitler DF, Amendola A, Bailey CS, et al. Posterior ankle arthroscopy: an anatomic study. J Bone Joint Surg Am 2002;84A(5):763–9.
15. Siddiqui MA, Chong KW, Yeo W, et al. Subtalar arthroscopy using a 2.4-mm zero-degree arthroscope: indication, technical experience, and results. Foot Ankle Spec 2010;3(4):167–71.
16. Williams MM, Ferkel RD. Subtalar arthroscopy: indications, technique, and results. Arthroscopy 1998;14(4):373–81.
17. Frey C, Feder KS, DiGiovanni C. Arthroscopic evaluation of the subtalar joint: does sinus tarsi syndrome exist? Foot Ankle Int 1999;20(3):185–91.

18. Horibe S, Kita K, Natsu-ume T, et al. A novel technique of arthroscopic excision of a symptomatic os trigonum. Clin Orthop Relat Res 2008;24:121–4.

19. Rammelt S, Gavlik JM, Barthel S, et al. The Value of Subtalar Arthroscopy in the Management of Intra-articular Calcaneus Fractures. Foot Ankle Int 2002;23(10): 906–16.

20. Sitte W, Lampert C, Baumann P. Osteosynthesis of talar body shear fractures assisted by hindfoot and subtalar arthroscopy: technique tip. Foot Ankle Int 2012; 33(1):74–8.

21. Glanzmann M, Sanhueza-Hernandez R. Arthroscopic subtalar arthrodesis for symptomatic osteoarthritis of the hindfoot: a prospective study of 41 cases. Foot Ankle Int 2007;28(1):2–7.

22. Albert A, Deleu PA, Leemrijse T, et al. Posterior arthroscopic subtalar arthrodesis: ten cases at one-year follow-up. Orthop Traumatol Surg Res 2011;97(4):401–5.

23. Elgafy H, Ebraheim NA. Subtalar arthroscopy for persistent subfibular pain after calcaneal fractures. Foot Ankle Int 1999;20(7):422–7.

24. Oloff LM, Schulhofer SD, Bocko AP. Subtalar joint arthroscopy for sinus tarsi syndrome: a review of 29 cases. J Foot Ankle Surg 2001;40(3):152–7.

Hallux Metatarsophalangeal Arthroscopy: Indications and Techniques

Alberto Siclari, MD[a],*, Marco Piras, MD[b]

KEYWORDS

- Arthroscopy • Hallux metatarsophalangeal joint • Hallux valgus • Hallux rigidus
- Arthrodesis

KEY POINTS

- Arthroscopy of the first metatarsophalangeal joint requires an experienced surgeon with arthroscopy skills.
- Many patients with pathologic conditions involving the hallux can be treated with an arthroscopic procedure, with good long-term outcomes comparable to those with open surgery, but with lower postoperative pain and complications.
- Frequently this procedure is only a part of the treatment of hallux disorders and should be considered within the management algorithm.

HISTORY

Wanatabe[1] first described arthroscopic treatment of the first metatarsophalangeal joint in 1972. Bartlett[2] first reported its use in 1988. Ferkel and Van Breuken[3] were the first to present their technique and results in a series of patients in 1991. In 2006, Debnath and colleagues[4] noted 95% of patients remained pain-free at 2 years after first metatarsophalangeal joint (MTPJ) arthroscopy for treatment of early signs of degenerative joint disease. In 2008, Lui[5] demonstrated a statistically significant correlation between joint cartilage erosion, joint synovitis, and pain in hallux valgus. He also noted a statistically significant correlation between the size of cartilage defect and severity of hallux valgus using diagnostic arthroscopy of the first MTPJ. In 2009, Wang and colleagues[6] noted a statistically significant decrease in recurrence of acute gouty arthritis to the first MTPJ after arthroscopic debridement of tophi when compared with patients treated by medical means alone. Lui[7] reported on performing

The authors has nothing to disclose.
[a] Orthopedic Department, Nuovo Ospedale degli Infermi, St Cantone Rondolina 50, Biella, ASLBI, Piemonte 13900, Italy; [b] Orthopedic Department, Nuovo Ospedale degli Infermi, Ponderano, Biella, ASLBI, Piemonte 13875, Italy
* Corresponding author.
E-mail address: alsicl@libero.it

Foot Ankle Clin N Am 20 (2015) 109–122
http://dx.doi.org/10.1016/j.fcl.2014.10.012
1083-7515/15/$ – see front matter © 2015 Elsevier Inc. All rights reserved.

arthroscopy on the great toe joint for hallux valgus deformity, with good results. Siclari and Decantis[8] described combined treatment of hallux valgus deformity with arthroscopy and percutaneous distal osteotomy in 2009.

GROSS AND ARTHROSCOPIC ANATOMY

As with any surgical procedure, a firm understanding of the anatomy of the first MTPJ is required to perform arthroscopy.[9] In describing the first MTPJ complex, the base of the proximal phalanx of the hallux is ovoid in shape, wider than it is tall, and concave medial to lateral and dorsal to plantar. Little stability is gained from the chondral shape of the first MTPJ, because of the shallow articulation between the phalanx and the metatarsal head.[10] The rounded head of the first metatarsal has a side-to-side curvature that is greater than the vertical curvature and is somewhat wider (20–24 mm) than its height (16–20 mm).[11] The articular surface, covered by hyaline cartilage, extends onto the dorsal aspect of the metatarsal head and continues plantarly into the medial and lateral grooves, which serve as articulations for the sesamoid bones, with the medial groove larger and deeper to accommodate for the larger tibial sesamoid. The plantar grooves are separated by a median crest, known as the *crista*.[11] The joint capsule of the first MTPJ attaches close to cartilaginous edges dorsally; however, plantarly it attaches several millimeters proximal to the cartilage, with the plantar aspect of the capsule thicker than the dorsal capsule because of the presence of the plantar metatarsophalangeal ligament. The metatarsosesamoid ligaments thicken the medial and lateral aspects of the joint capsule, along with the medial and lateral collateral ligaments, which tract from the medial and lateral metatarsal tubercles to the corresponding tubercles on the sides of the phalanx.[11] The sesamoid bones of the flexor hallucis brevis muscle are attached to the metatarsal via the metatarsosesamoid ligaments and to the proximal phalanx of the hallux via the phalangeal sesamoid ligaments. The sesamoids also firmly adhere to the plantar metatarsophalangeal ligament, which results in a firm attachment to the proximal phalanx. The sesamoids therefore do not move relative to the proximal phalanx, but rather move relative to the metatarsal. Along with the ligamentous attachments already described, there are also tendon attachments to the sesamoid bones. The tibial sesamoid provides an insertion point for the abductor hallucis, and the fibular sesamoid provides an insertion point for the adductor hallucis and the deep transverse metatarsal ligament (**Fig. 1**).

The articular surface of the base of the first metatarsal is 25 to 30 mm deep and 16 to 20 mm wide, and the surface is concave dorsally and flat or slightly convex in the more plantar aspect of the joint.[12]

Intra-articular examination includes visualization of 10 major areas: the lateral gutter, the lateral corner of the metatarsal head, the central portion of the metatarsal head, the medial corner of the metatarsal head, the medial gutter, the medial portion of the proximal phalanx, the central portion of the proximal phalanx, the lateral portion of the proximal phalanx, the medial sesamoid, and the lateral sesamoid.

BIOMECHANICS

Biomechanically, the instant centers of motion for the first MTP joint are located within the metatarsal head. Motion occurs between the metatarsal head and the proximal phalanx via a sliding action at the joint surface. In full extension or flexion, this sliding action gives way to compression of the dorsal or plantar articular surfaces of the metatarsal head and the proximal phalanx.[13] Active range of motion of the hallux MTPJ in dorsiflexion averages 51° and 23° in plantar flexion. Additional passive range of motion in dorsiflexion averages 23°. In the hallux interphalangeal joint, the active flexion averages 46° and extension 12°, with additional passive dorsiflexion of 22°.[10]

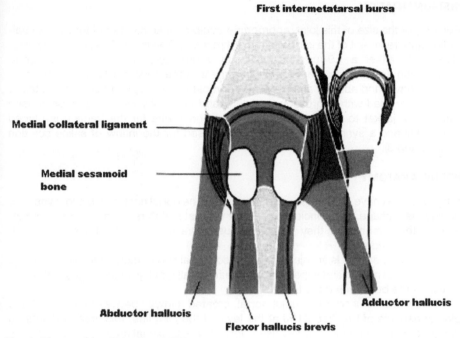

Fig. 1. Plantar side of the first MTPJs.

INDICATIONS

The advantages of arthroscopic treatment include minimal soft tissue dissection, avoiding a large capsulotomy, decreased postoperative pain, and less postoperative stiffness, with an improved outcome in selected groups of patients with symptomatic first MTPJ disease.

Primary indications for the MTPJ arthroscopy include

- Hallux rigidus
- Hallux valgus
- Synovitis
- Loose bodies
- Arthrofibrosis

Contraindications include the presence of large osteophytes that prevent adequate visualization of the anatomy, severe swelling, arterial insufficiency, soft tissue infection, and soft tissue compromise.

PREOPERATIVE PLANNING

Standard radiographic evaluation with standing views of the foot is essential for a correct diagnosis. A complete examination includes anteroposterior, lateral, and oblique views. A tangential view of the sesamoids can visualize the metatarsosesamoid articulation. Evaluation of radiographs can identify signs of arthritis, including joint space narrowing and osteophyte formation. MRI or computer tomography scanning may be useful in determining the presence of focal osteochondral defects or other associated pathologies.[10]

INSTRUMENTATION

Because of the size of this joint, appropriate equipment is mandatory for both visualization and treatment of the joint with the arthroscope. The first MTPJ is typically visualized with either a 1.9-mm or a 2.3-mm arthroscope, which allows for good visualization and enough room for the treatment of the abnormality within this joint. A small shaver and abrader also are used for most arthroscopic procedures. A tester is frequently used with arthroscopic pincers, and frequently the arthroscope is used without the jacket to reduce the obstruction. The k-wire for the traction is placed with a drill and a syringe with a connector is used for the inflow of saline solution (**Figs. 2** and **3**).

PORTAL ANATOMY

Surgeons must have a thorough understanding of the portal anatomy to avoid vascular or nervous damage. The principal portals for the first metatarsal joint are the dorsolateral and the dorsomedial; they are created just lateral and medial to the extensor hallucis longus tendon.

The possible danger is an injury to the dorsomedial and dorsolateral hallucal nerves (deep peroneal medial and superficial peroneal lateral) that lay on the edges of the projection of the bone with the artery.

A third portal is used, the medial portal, created midway between the dorsal and plantar aspects of the first MTPJ at the level of the joint line; this area presents no danger of nerve damage. A rarely used portal is the proximal medial portal between the abductor hallucis tendon and the medial head of the flexor hallucis brevis (**Fig. 4**).

SURGICAL TECHNIQUE
Step 1

The patient is placed in the supine position and several different types of anesthesia may be administered, including a regional block and general anesthesia. The use of a tourniquet is optional and may depend on the extent of the procedure.[10]

Step 2

To obtain sufficient visualization during this procedure, distraction is needed to increase the working articular space. A common technique is distraction using a

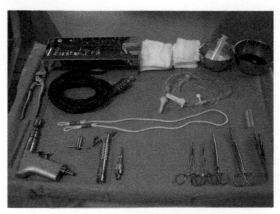

Fig. 2. Instrumentation: traction, manual pump, and drill.

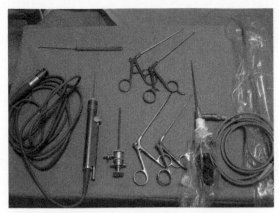

Fig. 3. Instrumentation: arthroscope, drill, and arthroscopic pincers.

Chinese finger trap with traction of 2 kg over a pulley attached to the surgical table. This procedure has some detriments: during the scope, the moisture from the portals may cause the hallux to slip out of the finger trap, resulting in a possible iatrogenic cartilage injury; in addition, the size of the finger trap may encumber the normal surgical operations. In the second distraction technique, the hallux is suspended using a Kirschner wire in the distal phalanx from an articulated arm on the operating table; the weight of the foot itself produces the distraction. This method is simple and no complications have been recorded in the distal phalanx (**Figs. 5** and **6**).[8]

Step 3

The dorsomedial portal is first established (**Fig. 7**). With a 14-gauge needle and 3 to 4 mL of saline solution, the joint is injected to confirm adequate placement; than a second 14-gauge needle is placed in the dorsolateral portal. The saline flow indicates the correct position (**Fig. 8**).

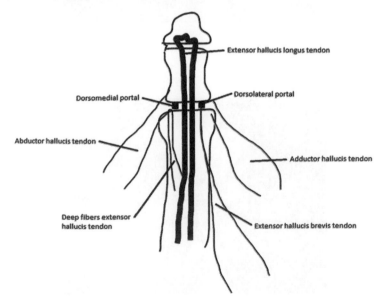

Extensor hallucis longus tendon

Dorsomedial portal

Dorsolateral portal

Abductor hallucis tendon

Adductor hallucis tendon

Deep fibers extensor hallucis tendon

Extensor hallucis brevis tendon

Fig. 4. The dorsal portals.

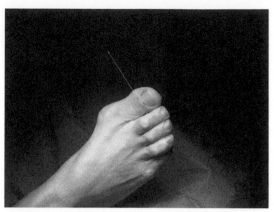

Fig. 5. Position of the K-wire for traction.

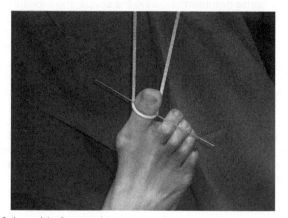

Fig. 6. Position of the cable for traction.

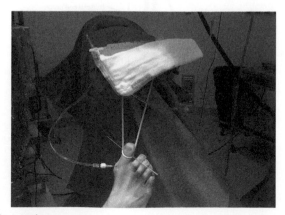

Fig. 7. The foot in traction.

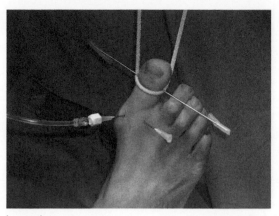

Fig. 8. The 2 dorsal portals.

Step 4

A mini longitudinal incision is made following the lateral needle. A mosquito forceps is used to spread the soft tissue to allow insertion of a 1.9-mm arthroscope (**Figs. 9** and **10**). In this procedure, the arthroscopic portal must be changed from medial to lateral frequently so that the inflow is positioned with a plantar needle placed at the medial portal (**Fig. 11**).

Step 5

A pump system may be used to provide low-pressure flow, but it is possible to use only a syringe handled by an assistant, because this technique is a low-demanding pressure procedure.

Step 6: Special Techniques

Hallux rigidus

This arthroscopic technique is possible for treating hallux rigidus only in the first 2 stages (**Fig. 12**).

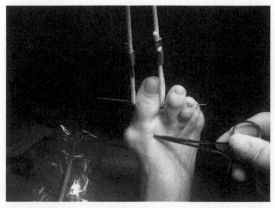

Fig. 9. The mosquito operation.

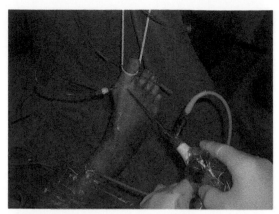

Fig. 10. The use of the lateral portal.

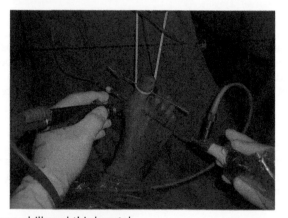

Fig. 11. Arthroscope, drill, and third portal.

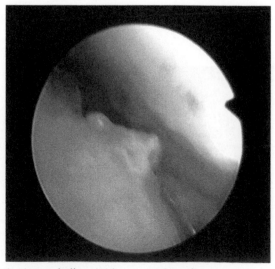

Fig. 12. Arthroscopic view: a hallux rigidus, second grade.

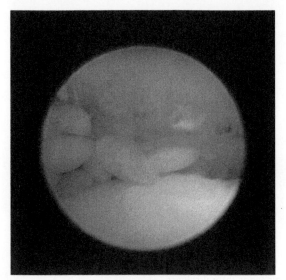

Fig. 13. Arthroscopic view: synovial hypertrophy.

The goal is to perform a cheilectomy to improve the hallux movement. To perform this procedure, a shaver is positioned orthogonal to the first metatarsal axis to remove the spurs, alternatively from the dorsolateral and dorsomedial portal.

Technical tip In the first part of this procedure it is better to use a shaver for the soft tissue and then use a shaver for the bone.

Hallux valgus
The arthroscope is used to shave the synovial hypertrophy (**Figs. 13** and **14**) and perform a distal soft tissue release. In this release, the lateral-inferior capsule and

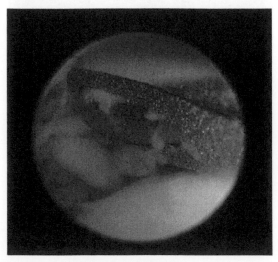

Fig. 14. Arthroscopic view: synovectomy with shaver.

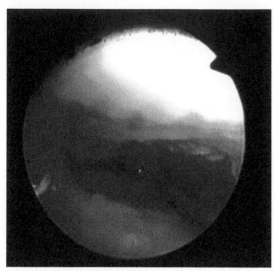

Fig. 15. Arthroscopic view: lateral release.

the abductor tendon must be cut (**Figs. 15** and **16**). The arthroscopic portion is only an initial step of the procedure.

Technical tip It is easier, and safer, to use an arthroscopic blade (eg, a micro-banana blade) to perform this procedure (**Fig. 17**).

Synovitis
The arthroscope is used to assist the soft shaver to perform a correct synovectomy (**Fig. 18**).

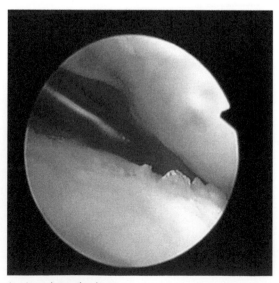

Fig. 16. Arthroscopic view: lateral release.

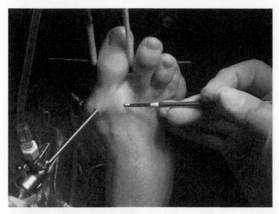

Fig. 17. Arthroscopic view: arthroscopic blade.

Technical tip It is beneficial for hemostasis to use a higher-flow system, and therefore use of the pump system or gravity is recommended.

Loose bodies

As with other joints, arthroscopic removal of loose bodies is one of the best indications for using a scope. These objects are osteochondral fragments or foreign bodies, and an arthroscopic pincer is used (**Fig. 19**).

Technical tip Use a low-inflow system to reduce the movement of the loose body.

Arthrofibrosis

Arthrofibrosis is a rare condition characterized by a loss of mobility caused by a fibrosis of the capsule (**Fig. 20**). The goal of this procedure is to "thin" the capsular attachment to make the hallux more elastic.

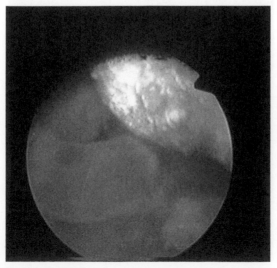

Fig. 18. Arthroscopic view: synovitis.

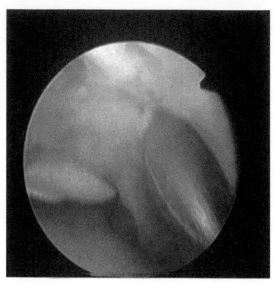

Fig. 19. Arthroscopic view: a loose body on the left.

Technical tip It is easier to use a nonaggressive soft shaver to avoid completely removing the capsule.

Arthrodesis

Arthrodesis is indicated for advanced stages of hallux rigidus, and for failed hallux valgus surgeries. The goal is to remove all the cartilage and prepare the subchondral surfaces to permit an arthrodesis with 2 percutaneous screws.

Technical tip To denude the cartilage completely, it is better to use all 3 portals with the shaver.

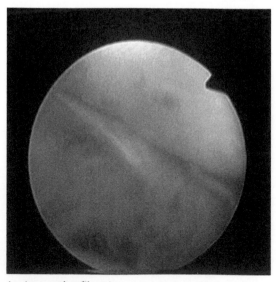

Fig. 20. Arthroscopic view: arthrofibrosis.

Box 1
Complications of the first metatarsophalangeal arthroscopy

1. Neurovascular injury near the portals

2. Plantar vascular injury during the distal tissue release

3. Vascular injury during a cheilectomy: dorsal arteries for the metatarsal head

4. Excessive capsular removal

5. Loss of traction system (Chinese finger trap)

6. Articular placement (interphalangeal) of the K-wire

Step 7: General Technical Tip

At the end of the procedure, local anesthesia with a long-duration drug, such as levobupivacaine, is recommended to reduce a postsurgical pain for 6 to 7 hours.

Arthroscopy complications

The reported complications for this procedure are rare if the surgeon uses correct technique. The main risks for the procedure are listed in **Box 1**. The procedure-related complications include nerve or vascular injury from poorly placed portals, iatrogenic articular cartilage injury, inadequate fluid management, compartment ischemia, infections, effusion after surgery, and complex regional pain syndrome. The general complications are rare. One possible complication is damage to the arthroscope in the proximal connection, because of the fragility of this part. The authors maintain that this is a surgeon complication, not a patient complication.

Postoperative care

The postoperative care is dictated by the diagnosis and surgery performed; a patient who has undergone a simple arthroscopic synovectomy may weight-bear as tolerated while wearing a postoperative shoe. After an arthrodesis, many surgeons restrict weight-bearing for several days to weeks.

SUMMARY

Arthroscopic management of the first metatarsophalangeal joint is a specialized technique, and should not be performed by the occasional arthroscopist. If performed for the right indications and with the correct technique, this procedure has a favorable outcome with minimal complications.

REFERENCES

1. Watanabe M. Selfoc-Arthroscope (Watanabe no. 24 arthroscope). Monograph. Tokyo: Teishin Hospital; 1972. p. 46–53.

2. Bartlett DH. Arthroscopic management of osteochondritis dissecans of the first metatarsal head. Arthroscopy 1988;4(1):51–4.

3. Ferkel RD, Van Breuken KP. Great toe arthroscopy: indications, technique, and results. Presented at the Annual Meeting of the Arthroscopy Association of North America. San Diego, May 6, 1991.

4. Debnath UK, Hemmady MV, Hariharan K. Indications for and technique of first MTP arthroscopy. Foot Ankle Int 2006;27(12):1049–54.

5. Lui TH. First metatarsophalangeal joint arthroscopy in patients with hallux valgus. Arthroscopy 2008;24(10):1122–9.

6. Wang CC, Lien SB, Huang GS, et al. Arthroscopic elimination of monosodium urate deposition of the first metatarsophalangeal joint reduces the recurrence of gout. Arthroscopy 2009;25(2):153–8.

7. Lui TH. Metatarsophalangeal joint arthroscopy in patients with hallux valgus. Arthroscopy 2008;24(10):1122–9.

8. Siclari A, Decantis V. Arthroscopic lateral release and percutaneous distal osteotomy for hallux valgus: a preliminary report. Foot Ankle Int 2009;30(7):675–9.

9. Derner R, Naldo J. Small joint arthroscopy of the foot. Clin Podiatr Med Surg 2011;28:551–60.

10. Carreira DS. Arthroscopy of the hallux. Foot Ankle Clin N Am 2009;14:105–14.

11. Hirsch BE, Minugh-Purvis N. Anatomy of the lower extremity. Philadelphia: Elsevier; 2005.

12. Faure C. The skeleton of the anterior foot. Anat Clin 1981;3:49–65.

13. Frey C, van Dijk CN. Arthroscopy of the great toe. Instr Course Lect 1999;48:343–6.

Small Joint Arthroscopy in Foot and Ankle

Tun Hing Lui, MBBS (HK), FRCS (Edin), FHKAM, FHKCOS[a],*,
Chi Pan Yuen, MBBS (HK), FRCS (Edin), FHKAM[b]

KEYWORDS

- Metatarsophalangeal joint • Interphalangeal joint • Lisfranc joint • Chopart joint
- Tarsometatarsal

KEY POINTS

- The techniques of small joint arthroscopy of the foot and ankle are rapidly evolving.
- The indications of small joint arthroscopy range from simple synovectomy to complex reconstructive procedures.
- Safety and efficacy of small joint arthroscopy need to be determined by further study.

METATARSOPHALANGEAL JOINT OF THE LESSER TOES
Anatomy

The metatarsophalangeal (MTP) joint of the lesser toe consists of the articulation between the metatarsal head and the proximal phalanx. The bony architecture conformity is minimal compared with the MTP-1. Therefore, the lesser MTP joint is stabilized primarily by the plantar plate; medial and lateral collateral ligaments; joint capsule; and traversing tendons.[1] The plantar plate arises from the metatarsal head just proximal to the articular surface and inserts on the base of the proximal phalanx. The collateral ligaments are composed of 2 bands: the phalangeal collateral ligament, which inserts onto the base of the proximal phalanx, and the accessory collateral ligament, which inserts onto the plantar plate.[2]

General Arthroscopic Technique

Positioning
The patient is placed in a supine position. A thigh tourniquet is applied to provide a bloodless surgical field. The surgeon is seated at the lateral side of the operated foot with the monitor at the end of the bed.

There is no conflict of interest in preparation of this article.
[a] Department of Orthopaedics and Traumatology, North District Hospital, 9 Po Kin Road, Sheung Shui, NT, Hong Kong 999077, China; [b] Department of Orthopaedics and Traumatology, Kwong Wah Hospital, 25 Waterloo Road, Hong Kong 999077, China
* Corresponding author.
E-mail address: luithderek@yahoo.co.uk

Foot Ankle Clin N Am 20 (2015) 123–138
http://dx.doi.org/10.1016/j.fcl.2014.10.007
1083-7515/15/$ – see front matter © 2015 Elsevier Inc. All rights reserved.

foot.theclinics.com

Traction

Manual traction is usually sufficient for intra-articular visualization and instrumentation. Instrumented traction is not used routinely because at the time of opening up the joint space, it makes the intra-articular gutters obliterated and decreases the maneuverability of the arthroscope and instruments.

Instruments

A 1.9-mm 30° small joint arthroscope is used. Gravity-driven inflow is always adequate.

Portals

Commonly used portals are the dorsomedial and dorsolateral portals.

The dorsomedial and dorsolateral portals are at the level of joint line medial and lateral to the extensor digitorum longus tendon. The dorsal digital branches of superficial peroneal nerve are at risk because they are in close proximity to the portals.

Arthroscopic examination

The portal sites are located with a 21-gauge needle before skin incision. The subcutaneous tissue is bluntly dissected with a hemostat and the joint capsule is perforated by the tip of the hemostat. The capsular opening should not be enlarged by spreading of the hemostat. The portals are interchangeable as visualization and instrumentation portals. The articular cartilage of the metatarsal head and the proximal phalanx is examined for chondral lesions. The plantar plate can be probed for any tear with manual distraction of the joint. The collateral ligaments can be seen at the medial and lateral gutters of the joint. Finally, the dorsal capsule can be examined by rotating the arthroscope toward the dorsum of the foot.

Specific Arthroscopic Technique

Arthroscopic synovectomy

Common causes for MTP synovitis include metabolic (eg, gouty arthritis), inflammatory (eg, rheumatoid arthritis), infection, and abnormal mechanical stress (eg, hallux valgus).[3–6] Arthroscopic synovectomy is indicated for pain and swelling control once conservative treatment fails.

Technique
1. To avoid crowding of instruments during a synovectomy of the dorsal gutter, the portals can be spaced slightly farther from the extensor tendons.
2. Synovectomy of the medial gutter can be done with the arthroscope at the dorsolateral portal and the arthroscopic shaver at the dorsomedial portal and vice versa for synovectomy of the lateral gutter.
3. Synovectomy of the plantar gutter is always possible by manual traction of the joint (**Fig. 1**).

Arthroscopic-assisted double plantar plate tenodesis for metatarsophalangeal instability

Claw toe deformity is the most common lesser toe deformity. The key component of this deformity is hyperextension of the MTP joint.[7,8] The primary pathology is at the plantar plate, which is attenuated at the attachment over the metatarsal neck, leading to distal and dorsal subluxation.[9,10] Finally, the proximal synovial attachment ruptures and the MTP joint dislocates.[11]

Surgical correction with soft tissue and bony surgical procedures has been described in cases of failed conservative management. The most common soft tissue procedure is a flexor to extensor tendon transfer. It works as a static tenodesis and a

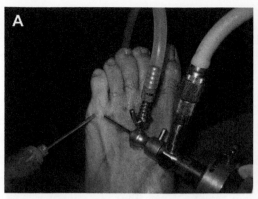
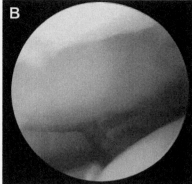

Fig. 1. (A) MTP arthroscopy of the fifth toe. (B) Arthroscopic synovectomy of the plantar recess through dorsal portals.

stiff toe is a common complication. Shortening osteotomies (eg, Weil osteotomy), excisional arthroplasty, and arthrodesis are common bony procedures for severe deformities. Postoperative stiffness, however, is also common.[11–16] Direct repair of the plantar plate has been proposed to decrease postoperative toe stiffness.[9,17,18]

Arthroscopic-assisted plantar plate tenodesis[19–21] can tackle the primary pathology of plantar plate attenuation. It stabilizes the plantar plate by suturing the plantar plate to the long extensor tendon with a figure-of-eight configuration. The pull of the extensor tendon redirects plantarly to stabilize the plantar plate. This technique is best indicated if the plantar plate is disrupted at the metatarsal side. It still works, however, if the plantar plate is disrupted at the phalangeal insertion because the stitch is holding the plantar plate–fibrous flexor tendon sheath complex rather than the plantar plate alone. The role of arthroscopy is to detect and treat any concomitant intra-articular pathology and assess the status of the plantar plate. The insertion of the needle through the plantar plate can be guided arthroscopically if there are tears at the plate (**Fig. 2**).

Technique
1. MTP arthroscopy is performed with 2 portals, dorsomedial and dorsolateral. The plantar plate is examined and any concomitant intra-articular pathology is treated.
2. The dorsal capsule is stripped from the metatarsal neck with a small periosteal elevator.
3. A PDS 1 suture is passed through the lateral part of the plantar plate with a straight-eyed needle through the dorsolateral portal with the arthroscope at the dorsomedial portal.
4. The needle is pierced through the plantar plate–fibrous flexor tendon sheath complex and the plantar skin. The MTP joint of the toe is flexed during the passage of the needle.
5. A second dorsal longitudinal incision is made at the diaphysis of the metatarsal. A curved hemostat is introduced at the medial side of the metatarsal directed toward the plantar aspect of distal metatarsal, deep to the flexor tendons, and then to the plantar lateral side of the fibrous tendon sheath. The suture is retrieved through the proximal wound.
6. The second limb of the suture is passed from the dorsolateral portal toward the dorsomedial portal and then passed through the medial part of the plantar plate by means of a straight-eyed needle. The suture is retrieved along the lateral side of the metatarsal to the proximal wound.

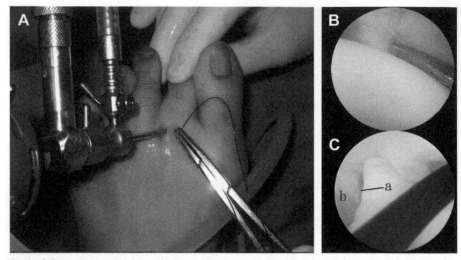

Fig. 2. (*A*) Arthroscopic-assisted plantar plate tenodesis. (*B*) The suture is passed through the plantar plate by means of a straight-eyed needle under arthroscopic guidance. (*C*) With visualization using the scope, the suture is passed through the intact part of the plantar plate which is away from the tear of the plantar plate (a). Flexor digitorum longus tendon that was exposed through the tear of the plantar plate (b).

7. The suture is secured to the extensor digitorum longus tendon at the proximal dorsal wound.
8. The suture is tensioned with the ankle kept in neutral position, so that the affected MTP joint is reduced spontaneously, and the suture is tied over the long extensor tendon.
9. The procedure is repeated and 2 figure-of-eight configuration of sutures connecting plantar plate–flexor tendon sheath complex to extensor digitorum longus are constructed.
10. Postoperatively, patients are allowed to walk with a hard bottom postoperative shoe and toe mobilization is allowed.

Arthroscopic interpositional arthroplasty for Freiberg infarction

Smillie[22] divided the clinical progress of Freiberg disease into 5 stages. A closing wedge osteotomy has been proposed to decompress the joint.[23] A pattern of arthroscopic management of this disease was outlined by Carro and colleagues.[24] Arthroscopic removal of loose body and débridement is recommended in early stages of all age groups. Arthroscopic osteochondral transplantation should be considered in late adolescence or early adulthood with late disease. An arthroscopic Keller procedure is reserved as salvage procedure in the later stages (stages IV and V).

el-Tayeby[25] described an interpositional arthroplasty for Freiberg disease. The tendon of the extensor digitorum longus is used for surfacing and as a joint spacer. The ability of the procedure to produce pain relief was satisfactory; however, the range of motion of the MTP joint did not improve. Arthroscopic interpositional arthroplasty[26] is indicated in adult patients with extensive involvement of the metatarsal head, especially when cartilage degeneration of the proximal phalanx is also present. This arthroscopic technique has the potential advantages of detailed examination and débridement of the joint while preserving the capsule and surrounding soft tissue. The use of extensor digitorum brevis tendon as the interpositional material can preserve the extensor digitorum longus tendon and active extension of the toe. Tendon interposition into the joint can facilitate the maintenance of joint space and prevent bone impingement during dorsiflexion/plantarflexion motion (**Fig. 3**).

Technique

1. MTP arthroscopy of the involved joint is performed with a dorsomedial and dorso-lateral portal on either side of extensor tendon.
2. Arthroscopic débridement of the damaged cartilage, synovectomy, and removal of loose body is performed.
3. The extensor digitorum brevis tendon is identified along the dorsolateral portal wound. The tendon is cut proximally through a proximal stab wound and is retrieved through the dorsolateral portal.
4. The tendon is rolled into a ball with a 3-0 Vicryl suture.
5. The stay stitch and the tendon ball are inserted into the joint by means of an eyed needle under arthroscopic guidance (**Fig. 4**).
6. The suture is passed through the plantar plate and plantar skin and is tied and cut flush to the plantar wound. Portal skin wounds are closed with 3-0 nylon.
7. Postoperatively, patients are allowed to walk with a hard bottom postoperative shoe and toe mobilization is allowed.

LISFRANC (TARSOMETATARSAL) JOINT

The tarsometatarsal joints (TMTJs) can be divided into 3 columns. The medial column consists of the first metatarsocuneiform joint. The middle column consists of the second and third metatarsocuneiform joints. The lateral column consists of the fourth and fifth metatarsocuboid joints.[27,28]

Joint stability is afforded through a combination of its bony architecture and ligamentous complex. In the coronal plane, the 3 cuneiforms, cuboid, and metatarsal bases

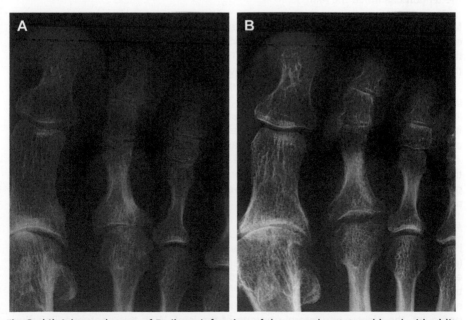

Fig. 3. (*A*) Advanced stage of Freiberg infarction of the second metatarsal head with obliteration of the joint space. (*B*) The joint space restored after arthroscopic interpositional arthroplasty.

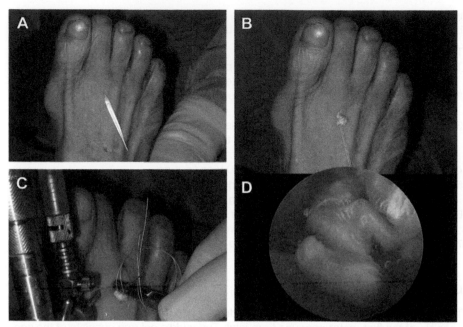

Fig. 4. Arthroscopic interpositional arthroplasty. (*A*) The extensor digitorum brevis tendon is identified at the dorsolateral portal wound. The tendon is cut proximally through a proximal stab wound and is retrieved to the dorsolateral portal. (*B*) The tendon is rolled into a ball with a 3.0-Vicryl suture. (*C*) The stay stitch and the tendon ball are inserted into the joint by means of an eyed needle under arthroscopic guidance. (*D*) Arthroscopic view shows the tendon ball inside the joint.

form the transverse arch of the midfoot, the so-called Roman arch configuration, which enhances stability. In the axial plane, the middle cuneiform is recessed proximally relative to the medial and lateral cuneiforms. This mortise configuration accommodates the base of the second metatarsal and provides additional osseous stability.[29]

The stability is further reinforced by the soft tissue ligamentous complex, which is grouped according to anatomic location (dorsal, plantar, and interosseous). The largest and strongest interosseous ligament is the Lisfranc ligament, which arises from the lateral surface of the medial cuneiform and inserts onto the medial aspect of the second metatarsal base near the plantar surface.[28]

Instability and posttraumatic arthritis are 2 common problems that can be treated through an arthroscopic tarsometatarsal arthrodesis.[30] Moreover, arthroscopic ganglionectomy[31] (**Fig. 5**) and arthrolysis[32] have also been reported to deal with ganglion and arthrofibrosis of those joints.

First Tarsometatarsal Instability

Hypermobility of the first TMTJ can be associated with different clinical pathologies (eg, hallux valgus, transfer metatarsalgia, and arthritis of the second TMTJ). Arthrodesis of the first TMTJ (modified Lapidus procedure) is indicated for symptomatic patients who fail nonoperative treatment.[33–35] An open procedure with a dorsomedial approach is associated with several complications due to the limited accessibility, in particular, the plantar and lateral portions of the joint. With this anatomic limitation, there is a tendency to remove excessive bone at the medial and dorsal parts of the joint, resulting in shortening and dorsal angulation or abduction of the first

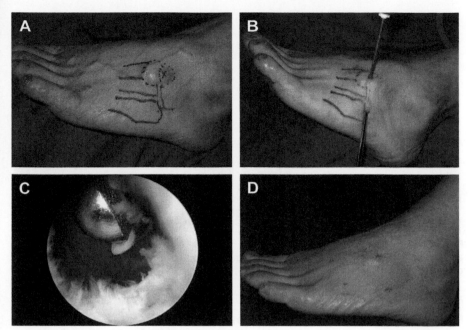

Fig. 5. (*A*) Ganglion arises from the Lisfranc joint. (*B*) Lisfranc arthroscopy with the P3-4 and lateral portals. (*C*) Arthroscopic ganglionectomy. (*D*) Excellent cosmetic results after the operation.

metatarsal.[33] The arthroscopic Lapidus procedure has the advantage of better visualization of the deep part of the joint, more thorough preparation of the fusion site with less bone removal, and reduced risk of malunion or nonunion.[36,37] Occasionally, this can be used as a revision arthrodesis for symptomatic first metatarsocuneiform nonunion after open Lapidus procedure.[38]

Technique
1. Patients are supine with a thigh tourniquet. A 2.7-mm 30° arthroscope is used.
2. Two portals are established at the plantar medial and dorsomedial corners of the joint.
3. The joint is identified by moving the first metatarsal and locating the motion at the first TMTJ and the portals are confirmed with a 22-gauge needle before incision. The position of the needle can be checked under fluoroscopy if needed.
4. The articular cartilage is denuded by an arthroscopic osteotome, exposing the subchondral bone. The subchondral bone is then microfractured by an arthroscopic awl (**Fig. 6**).
5. The intermetatarsal angle is closed up manually and the first metatarsal is plantarflexed by dorsiflexion of the first MTPJ. The degree of plantarflexion should be titrated so that there would not be excessive pressure under the first or second metatarsals.
6. A 4.0-mm cannulated screw is inserted from proximal dorsal to distal plantar direction across the joint. Finally, another 4.0-mm positional screw is inserted from the first metatarsal base to the second metatarsal base.
7. Postoperatively, patients are kept in an ankle-foot orthosis device and non–weight bearing. The positional screw is removed at 12 weeks.

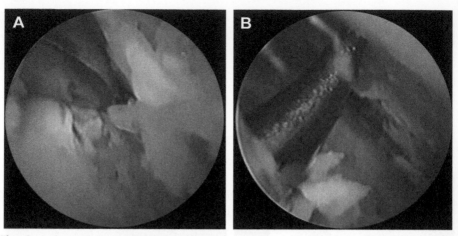

Fig. 6. Arthroscopic Lapidus arthrodesis. (*A*) Articular cartilage is denuded with a small arthroscopic osteotome leaving the subchondral bone intact. (*B*) Microfracture of the subchondral bone with an arthroscopic awl.

Posttraumatic Arthritis

Posttraumatic arthritis is the most common complication after a TMTJ injury, but not all patients with arthritic changes are symptomatic.[39] Kuo and colleagues[40] reported that 12 of 48 patients (25%) had symptomatic arthritis at final follow-up. Of these, 6 underwent open arthrodesis. Overall, the results of arthrodesis for posttraumatic arthritis are fair to average.[27,39]

One cadaveric study[41] had shown that the motion in the medial and middle columns is minimal, whereas most of the midfoot movement occurs in the lateral column. With increased loads, the articular contact forces increase significantly over the medial and middle columns but not the lateral column. This may partly explain why arthritic conditions less frequently involve the lateral column.

Six portals have been described for an arthroscopic tarsometatarsal arthrodesis. The choice of the portals used depends on which columns are included in the fusion.

Technique
1. Patients are positioned supine with a thigh tourniquet. A 2.7-mm 30° arthroscope is used.
2. Six tarsometatarsal portals (medial, P1-2, P2-3, P3-4, P4-5, and lateral) are designed to approach the 5 tarsometatarsal articulations (**Fig. 7**). Apart from the medial and lateral portals, the other 4 portals are junction portals, with the capability of approaching the adjacent articulations. Moreover, these portals can be used to approach the intercuneiform spaces and spaces between the proximal parts of metatarsal bones. This can allow débridement and release of these spaces to facilitate reduction of the Lisfranc joint in both the sagittal and transverse planes.
   a. Medial portal: located at the plantar medial aspect of the first TMTJ. The first TMTJ can be approached with this portal.
   b. P1-2 portal: located at the junction point between the medial cuneiform, first metatarsal, and second metatarsal bones. The first TMTJ can be approached. The skin wound can be mobilized proximally to approach the second TMTJ.
   c. P2-3 portal: located at the junction point between the second metatarsal, intermediate cuneiform, and lateral cuneiform bones. The second TMTJ can be approached. The third TMTJ can be approached by moving the skin wound distally.

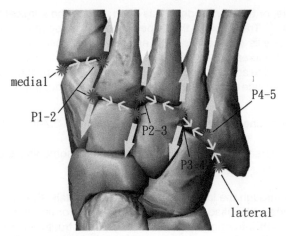

medial

P4-5

P1-2

P2-3

P3-4

lateral

Fig. 7. Illustration of the Lisfranc portals. The small, thin arrows show the joints approach by the individual portal. The wide arrows show the reach of the individual portal in longitudinal direction. Note that the P1-2 and P2-3 portals can be shifted in longitudinal direction to approach the adjacent joints.

    d. P3-4 portal: located at the junction point between lateral cuneiform, cuboid, third, and fourth metatarsal bones. The third and fourth TMTJs can be approached.

    e. P4-5 portal: located between the proximal articular surfaces of the fourth and fifth metatarsal bones. The fourth and fifth TMTJs can be approached.

    f. Lateral portal: located at the lateral corner of the fifth metatarsal-cuboid articulation. Besides the fifth metatarsal-cuboid articulation, the insertion of the peroneus brevis tendon and the peroneus tertius can also be approached through this portal.[32]

    g. The third, fourth, and fifth TMTJs share a common synovial lining and joint capsule and the joints are at the same level. Therefore, the P3-4, P4-5 and lateral portals are interchangeable to approach these 3 articulations.

3. Usually only the medial 3 TMTJs needed to be fused, unless there is recalcitrant pain over the fourth and fifth TMTJs. The corresponding joint spaces can be approached (as described previously). The fusion surfaces preparation technique is similar to arthroscopic Lapidus procedure. The 3 joints are reduced into desired position and transfixed with 4.0-mm cannulated screws. Cancellous bone graft can be packed into the fusion site through the portals with the aid of a small drill sleeve.

4. Postoperatively, patients are immobilized in a short leg cast with non—weight bearing for 8–12 weeks.

CHOPART (TRANSVERSE TARSAL) JOINT

The Chopart joint was named after Francois Chopart (1743–1795), who described the use of the talonavicular (TN) and calcaneocuboid (CC) articulations as a practical level for amputation.[42] It plays a critical role in allowing the foot to transition from a flexible structure when the hindfoot is in valgus during heel strike to a rigid structure when the hindfoot is in varus during toe-off.[43] Cadaveric studies have identified the pivotal biomechanical role of the TN joint for the hindfoot.[44]

    Causes of TN, CC, or subtalar joint arthritis can be posttraumatic, rheumatoid arthritis, or sequelae of pediatric foot deformities.

Isolated, double, or triple arthrodesis has been used in the surgical management of end-stage arthritis.[45] Traditionally, this is performed as an open procedure. Similar to other open arthrodesis procedures with extensive soft tissue dissection and bony resection, there is increased risk for pseudoarthrosis or nonunion.[46] Arthroscopic arthrodesis can provide an improved intra-articular visualization, minimal bone removal, and better fusion surface preparation. In theory, this can reduce the nonunion rate.[45]

Technique
1. Patients are positioned supine with a thigh tourniquet. A 2.7-mm 30° arthroscope is used.
2. There are 4 midtarsal portals: lateral, dorsolateral, dorsomedial, and medial portals (**Fig. 8**).
3. CC arthrodesis
   a. Performed through the lateral and dorsolateral portals (**Fig. 9**)[47]
   b. Lateral portal: identified at the plantar lateral corner of the CC joint and confirmed with intraoperative fluoroscopy. The structures at risk include the peroneal tendons and sural nerve.
   c. Dorsolateral portal: should be located under fluoroscopic guidance. It is directly over the space between the TN and CC joints. It is the most important portal of midtarsal arthroscopy because the medial aspect of the CC joint, the lateral and plantar aspects of the TN joint, the anterior subtalar joint, and the junction between the talus, calcaneus, navicular, and cuboid can be reached through this portal (**Fig. 10**). It can be used for arthroscopic resection of calcaneonavicular coalition or its variants[48] and the symptomatic nonunion of the anterior calcaneal process.[49] The lateral branch of superficial peroneal nerve and the lateral terminal branch of the deep peroneal nerve are at risk.[50,51]

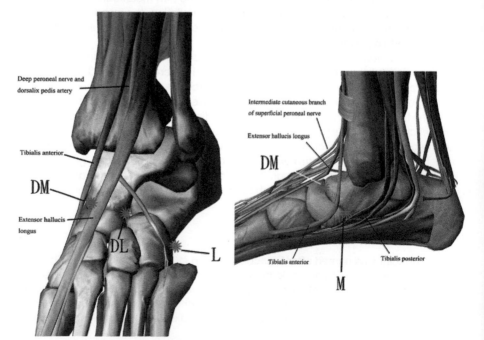

Fig. 8. Illustration of the midtarsal portals. DL, dorsolateral portal; DM, dorsomedial portal; L, lateral portal; M, medial portal.

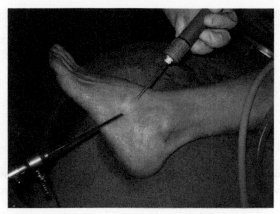

Fig. 9. CC arthroscopy with lateral and dorsolateral portals.

    d. These 2 portals are interchangeable as visualization and instrumentation portals.
4. TN arthrodesis
    a. Performed through the medial, dorsomedial, and dorsolateral portals.[46]
    b. Medial portal: located at the medial side of the TN joint, just dorsal to the posterior tibial tendon.
    c. Dorsomedial portal: located at the midpoint between the medial and dorsolateral portals. The intermediate cutaneous branch of superficial peroneal nerve and extensor hallucis longus tendon are at risk during creation of this portal.[47]
    d. The 3 portals are interchangeable as visualization and working portals (**Fig. 11**).
5. The fusion surface preparation, joint reduction, and fixation technique are similar to arthroscopic Lapidus procedure.
6. Postoperatively, patients are immobilized in a short leg cast and kept non–weight bearing for 8 weeks. After these restrictions, patients progress to protected weight bearing with rocker boot for another 4 weeks.

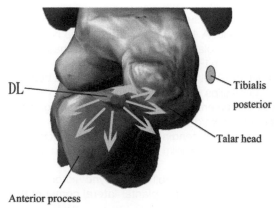

Fig. 10. Illustration of the areas reachable through the dorsolateral (DL) portal, including the medial aspect of the CC joint, the lateral and plantar aspects of the TN joint, the anterior subtalar joint, and the junction between the CC and TN joints.

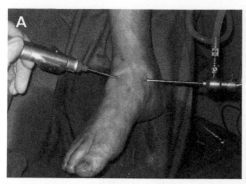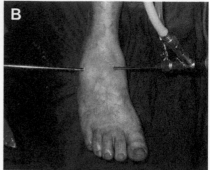

Fig. 11. TN arthroscopy. (A) Medial and dorsomedial portals. (B) Dorsomedial and dorsolateral portals.

Other indications for midtarsal arthroscopy include recalcitrant synovitis, ganglion cysts, and CC impingement. Moreover, the midtarsal joint functions together with the anterior and posterior subtalar joints. Anatomically, the TN joint shares the same capsule with the anterior subtalar joint. The midtarsal and subtalar arthroscopy, therefore, shares some of their portals and frequently work together. The portals and techniques of medial,[52,53] anterior,[54,55] and posterior subtalar arthroscopies are not discussed because they are beyond the scope of this article.

INTERPHALANGEAL ARTHROSCOPY OF THE TOES

Similar intra-articular pathologies (eg, osteoarthritis, synovitis, chondral lesion, arthrofibrosis, and instability) can occur in the interphalangeal (IP) joint of the toes as in other joints. Moreover, many corrective procedures of toe deformity involve excisional arthroplasty or arthrodesis of the IP joint.

IP arthroscopy of the toes has been described (**Fig. 12**). Among the various indications, arthroscopic ganglionectomy of recurrent IP ganglion is the single most described one.[56]

Technique
1. Patients are positioned in a supine position with a thigh pneumatic tourniquet to maintain a bloodless field. A 1.9-mm 30° arthroscope is used.
2. The dorsomedial and dorsolateral portal wounds are made at the dorsomedial and dorsolateral corners of the IP joint.
3. The portals of proximal IP arthroscopy should be placed between the collateral ligaments and the lateral slips of the tendon expansion.
4. The arthroscopic instruments should be inserted along the dorsal recess and should not be pointed toward the articular cartilage.
5. Visualization is obtained by extending and flexing the joint rather than trying to force the arthroscope into the narrow joint space. The joint can be distracted manually to improve the visual field.
6. A plantar lateral portal can be established if synovectomy of the plantar gutter is needed. The portal is located at the plantar lateral corner of the joint.

RESULTS

Most of the studies of small joint arthroscopy in foot and ankle are technical notes, case reports, or case series. No significant result can be concluded.

Study, Year of Publication	Design	Indication	Type of Arthroscopy	No. Cases (Procedures)	Mean Follow-up (mo)	Results
Lui,[55] 2010	Retrospective	Synovitis, osteoarthritis, claw toe deformity, recurrent ganglion, osteochondral lesion	IPJ	20 (22)	48	Heterogenous group of patients. Authors proposes that ganglion is the best indication for IP arthroscopy.
Carro et al,[24] 2004	Technical note	Freiberg disease	Lesser MTPJ	N/A	N/A	N/A
Lui,[26] 2007	Technical note	Freiberg disease	Lesser MTPJ	N/A	N/A	N/A
Lui,[20] 2007	Retrospective	Claw toe, overriding toe	Lesser MTPJ	13 (13)	6	Toe motion regained approximately 6 mo postoperative. One case of mild recurrence of transverse plane deformity
Lui et al,[35] 1992	Technical note	Hypermobility	TMTJ	N/A	N/A	N/A
Lui,[30] 2007	Technical note	Posttraumatic arthritis	TMTJ	N/A	N/A	N/A
Michels et al,[37] 2011	Retrospective	Hallux valgus with first TMTJ Hypermobility	TMTJ	5 (5)	12	Solid fusion in all the patients. The HVA improved by 25.6°. The IMA improved by 10.6°. Shortening of the first ray was limited to 2.7 mm.
Lui,[38] 2012	Technical note	Nonunion	TMTJ	N/A	N/A	N/A
Oloff et al,[47] 1996	Retrospective	Synovitis, osteoarthritis, osteochondral lesion	Transverse tarsal	7 (7)	7	Heterogenous group of patients. Five excellent and 2 good cases; 2 patients required arthrotomy.
Lui,[45] 2006	Technical note	Postpolio equinocavovarus deformity	Subtalar and transverse tarsal	N/A	N/A	N/A
Hammond et al,[51] 2011	Cadaveric	N/A	Transverse tarsal	N/A	N/A	N/A

Abbreviations: HVA, hallux valgus angle; IMA, intermetatarsal angle; IPJ, interphalangeal joint; N/A, not available.

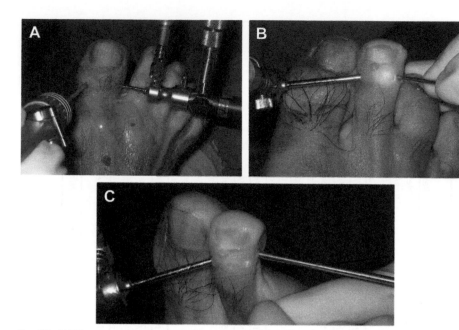

Fig. 12. (*A*) IP arthroscopy of the hallux. (*B*) Distal IP arthroscopy of the second toe with dorsomedial and dorsolateral portals. (*C*) Plantar lateral portal of the distal IP arthroscopy.

SUMMARY

Both the techniques and indications of small joint arthroscopies of the foot are rapidly evolving. Further study is needed, however, to evaluate their safety and efficacy.

REFERENCES

1. Sarrafian SK, Topouzian LK. Anatomy and physiology of the extensor apparatus of the toes. J Bone Joint Surg Am 1969;51:669–79.
2. Deland JT, Lee KT, Sobel M, et al. Anatomy of the plantar plate and its attachments in the lesser metatarsal phalangeal joint. Foot Ankle Int 1995;16:480–6.
3. Mann RA, Mizel MS. Monarticular nontraumatic synovitis of the metatarsophalangeal joint: a new diagnosis? Foot Ankle 1985;6:18–21.
4. Mizel MS, Michelson JD. Nonsurgical treatment of monarticular nontraumatic synovitis of the second metatarsophalangeal joint. Foot Ankle Int 1997;18:424–6.
5. Raunio P, Laine H. Synovectomy of the metatarsophalangeal joints in rheumatoid arthritis. Scand J Rheumatol 1987;16:12–7.
6. Vainio K. Morton's metatarsalgia in rheumatoid arthritis. Clin Orthop Relat Res 1979;142:85–9.
7. Frank GR, Johnson WM. The extensor shift procedure in the correction of clawtoe deformities in children. South Med J 1966;59:889–96.
8. Heyman CH. The operative treatment of clawfoot. J Bone Joint Surg 1932;14: 335–8.
9. Chalayon O, Chertman C, Guss AD, et al. Role of plantar plate and surgical reconstruction techniques on static stability of lesser metatarsophalangeal joints: a biomechanical study. Foot Ankle Int 2013;34:1436–42.
10. Peck CN, Macleod A, Barrie J. Lesser metatarsophalangeal instability: presentation, management, and outcomes. Foot Ankle Int 2012;33:565–70.

11. Green DR, Brekke M. Anatomy, biomechanics and pathomechanics of lesser digital deformities. Clin Podiatr Med Surg 1996;13:179–200.
12. Barbari SG, Brevig K. Correction of clawtoes by the Girdlestone–Taylor Xexor-extensor transfer procedure. Foot Ankle 1984;5:67–73.
13. Caterini R, Farsetti P, Tatantino U, et al. Arthrodesis of the toe joints with an intra-medullary cannulated screw for correction of hammertoe deformity. Foot Ankle Int 2004;25:256–61.
14. Karlock LG. Second metatarsophalangeal joint fusion: a new technique for cross-over hammertoe deformity. A preliminary report. J Foot Ankle Surg 2003;42:178–82.
15. Miller SJ. Hammer toe correction by arthrodesis of the proximal interphalangeal joint using a cortical bone allograft pin. J Am Podiatr Med Assoc 2002;92:563–9.
16. O'Kane C, Kilmartin T. Review of proximal interphalangeal joint excisional arthro-plasty for the correction of second hammer toe deformity in 100 cases. Foot Ankle Int 2005;26:320–5.
17. McAlister JE, Hyer CF. The direct plantar plate repair technique. Foot Ankle Spec 2013;6:446–51.
18. Nery C, Coughlin MJ, Baumfeld D, et al. Lesser metatarsophalangeal joint insta-bility: prospective evaluation and repair of plantar plate and capsular insuffi-ciency. Foot Ankle Int 2012;33:301–11.
19. Lui TH, Chan LK, Chan KB. Modified plantar plate tenodesis for correction of claw toe deformity. Foot Ankle Int 2010;31:584–91.
20. Lui TH. Arthroscopic-assisted correction of claw toe or overriding toe deformity: plantar plate tenodesis. Arch Orthop Trauma Surg 2007;127:823–6.
21. Lui TH. Stabilization of first metatarsophalangeal instability with plantar plate te-nodesis. J Foot Ankle Surg 2008;14:211–4.
22. Smillie IS. Treatment of Freiberg's infarction. Proc R Soc Med 1967;60:29–31.
23. Al-Ashhab ME, Kandel WA, Rizk AS. A simple surgical technique for treatment of Freiberg's disease. Foot 2013;23:29–33.
24. Carro LP, Golano P, Farinas O, et al. Arthroscopic Keller technique for Freiberg disease. Arthroscopy 2004;20:60–3.
25. el-Tayeby HM. Freiberg's infraction: a new surgical procedure. J Foot Ankle Surg 1998;27:23–7.
26. Lui TH. Arthroscopic interpositional arthroplasty for Freiberg's disease. Knee Surg Sports Traumatol Arthrosc 2007;15:555–9.
27. Komenda GA, Myerson MS, Biddinger KR. Results of arthrodesis of the tarsome-tatarsal joints after traumatic injury. J Bone Joint Surg Am 1996;78:1665–76.
28. de Palma L, Santucci A, Sabetta SP, et al. Anatomy of the Lisfranc joint complex. Foot Ankle Int 1997;18:356–64.
29. Thompson MC, Mormino MA. Injury to the tarsometatarsal joint complex. J Am Acad Orthop Surg 2003;11:260–7.
30. Lui TH. Arthroscopic tarsometatarsal (Lisfranc) arthrodesis. Knee Surg Sports Traumatol Arthrosc 2007;15:671–5.
31. Lui TH. Arthroscopic ganglionectomy of the foot and ankle. Knee Surg Sports Traumatol Arthrosc 2014;22(7):1693–700. http://dx.doi.org/10.1007/s00167-012-2065-8.
32. Lui TH. Lateral foot pain following open reduction and internal fixation of the frac-ture of the fifth metatarsal tubercle: treated by arthroscopic arthrolysis and endo-scopic tenolysis. BMJ Case Rep 2014;2014.
33. Lapidus PW. Operative correction of the metatarsus varus primus in hallux valgus. Surg Gynecol Obstet 1934;58:183–91.

34. Butson AR. A modification of Lapidus for hallux valgus. J Bone Joint Surg Br 1980;52:350–2.
35. Myerson MS. Metatarsocuneiform arthrodesis for management of hallux valgus and metatarsus primus varus. Foot Ankle 1992;13:107–15.
36. Lui TH, Chan KB, Ng S. Arthroscopic Lapidus arthrodesis. Arthroscopy 2005;21: 1516.
37. Michels F, Guillo S, de Lavigne C, et al. The arthroscopic Lapidus procedure. J Foot Ankle Surg 2011;17:25–8.
38. Lui TH. Symptomatic first metatarsocuneiform nonunion revised by arthroscopic lapidus arthrodesis. J Foot Ankle Surg 2012;51:656–9.
39. Myerson MS, Fisher RT, Burgess AR, et al. Fracture dislocations of the tarsometatarsal joints: end results correlated with pathology and treatment. Foot Ankle 1986;6:225–42.
40. Kuo RS, Tejwani NC, DiGiovanni CW, et al. Outcome after open reduction and internal fixation of Lisfranc joint injuries. J Bone Joint Surg Am 2000;82:1609–18.
41. Ouzounian TJ, Shereff MJ. In vitro determination of midfoot motion. Foot Ankle 1989;10:140–6.
42. Klaue K. Chopart fractures. Injury 2004;35:SB64–70.
43. Sammarco VJ. The talonavicular and calcaneocuboid joints: anatomy, biomechanics, and clinical management of the transverse tarsal joint. Foot Ankle Clin 2004;9:127–45.
44. Wulker N, Stukenborg C, Savory KM, et al. Hindfoot motion after isolated and combined arthrodeses: measurements in anatomic specimens. Foot Ankle Int 2000;21:921–7.
45. Lui TH. New technique of arthroscopic triple arthrodesis. Arthroscopy 2006;22: 464.e1–5.
46. Miehlke W, Gschwend N, Rippstein P, et al. Compression arthrodesis of the rheumatoid ankle and hindfoot. Clin Orthop 1997;340:75–86.
47. Oloff L, Schulhofer SD, Fanton G, et al. Arthroscopy of the calcaneocuboid and talonavicular joints. J Foot Ankle Surg 1996;35:101–8.
48. Lui TH. Arthroscopic resection of the calcaneonavicular coalition or the "too long" anterior process of the calcaneus. Arthroscopy 2006;22:903.e1–4.
49. Lui TH. Endoscopic excision of symptomatic nonunion of anterior calcaneal process. J Foot Ankle Surg 2011;50:476–9.
50. Lui TH, Chan LK. Safety and efficacy of talonavicular arthroscopy in arthroscopic triple arthrodesis. A cadaveric study. Knee Surg Sports Traumatol Arthrosc 2010; 18:607–11.
51. Hammond AW, Phisitkul P, Femino J, et al. Arthroscopic debridement of the talonavicular joint using dorsomedial and dorsolateral portals: a cadaveric study of safety and access. Arthroscopy 2011;27:228–34.
52. Lui TH, Chan LK, Chan KB. Medial subtalar arthroscopy: a cadaveric study of the tarsal canal portal. Knee Surg Sports Traumatol Arthrosc 2013;21:1279–82.
53. Lui TH. Medial subtalar arthroscopy. Foot Ankle Int 2012;33:1018–23.
54. Lui TH. Clinical tips: anterior subtalar (talocalcaneonavicular). Foot Ankle Int 2008;29:94–6.
55. Lui TH, Chan KB, Chan LK. Portal safety and efficacy of anterior subtalar arthroscopy: a cadaveric study. Knee Surg Sports Traumatol Arthrosc 2010;18:233–7.
56. Lui TH. Interphalangeal arthroscopy of the toes. Foot (Edinb) 2014;24:42–6.

Hindfoot Endoscopy for Posterior Ankle Impingement Syndrome and Flexor Hallucis Longus Tendon Disorders

Wataru Miyamoto, MD*, Masato Takao, MD, Takashi Matsushita, MD

KEYWORDS

- Hindfoot endoscopy • Posterior ankle impingement syndrome • Endoscopic surgery
- Flexor hallucis longus • Os trigonum • Stieda process

KEY POINTS

- Hindfoot endoscopy through a posterior 2-portal approach is an effective diagnostic and therapeutic procedure enabling direct visualization of posterior ankle pathology with low invasiveness.
- The most important point in hindfoot endoscopy for posterior ankle impingement syndrome and flexor hallucis longus (FHL) tendon disorders is identification at an early stage in surgery of the FHL tendon, which is located just lateral to the neurovascular bundle.
- After identifying the FHL tendon, the endoscopic procedure should be performed in the region lateral to the FHL tendon to avoid iatrogenic neurovascular injury.
- Although the occurrence of complications in hindfoot endoscopy is low, nerve injury especially to the sural or medial calcaneal nerve remains a common complication.

Videos of resections of the flexor hallucis longus tendon accompany this article at http://www.foot.theclinics.com/

INTRODUCTION

Since van Dijk and colleagues[1] introduced a 2-portal endoscopic approach for the diagnosis and treatment of posterior ankle pathology in 2000, hindfoot endoscopy has gained attention as a low-invasive procedure, and several surgical outcomes using this technique have been reported with good prognosis.[2–7] Hindfoot abnormalities

The authors have nothing to disclose.
Department of Orthopaedic Surgery, Teikyo University School of Medicine, 2-11-1 Kaga, Itabashi, Tokyo 173-8605, Japan
* Corresponding author.
E-mail address: miyamoto@med.teikyo-u.ac.jp

for which 2-portal hindfoot endoscopy is indicated include posterior ankle impingement syndrome (PAIS), FHL tendon disorder, and osteochondral lesions of the posterior tibiotalar or subtalar joint.[8,9]

Although no strict definition has been established, PAIS is typically considered a clinical disorder characterized by posterior ankle pain during forced plantar flexion,[8,9] and the most common causes of PAIS seem to be pathologic variants of the posterolateral talar process, such as an os trigonum (a nonfused secondary ossification center of the talus) and a Stieda process (a prominent posterolateral talar process).[8] These pathologic variants typically result from hyperplantarflexion of the ankle due to trauma or overuse. Furthermore, repetitive hyperflexion of the ankle can damage the posterior capsule, ligament, and synovium and thus also become a cause of PAIS.

FHL tendon disorder is another cause of posterior ankle pain.[8,9] The anatomic characteristic of an avascular zone of the FHL tendon existing behind the medial malleolus coupled with relative incongruency between the fibro-osseous tunnel and FHL tendon during full plantar and dorsiflexion of the ankle can easily cause chronic inflammation of the FHL tendon.[10,11] Hamilton and colleagues[10] reported an FHL tenosynovitis rate of 85% in dancers with posterior ankle pain, whereas Ogut and colleagues[6] reported that all 60 feet with posterior ankle pain in their series were accompanied by FHL tenosynovitis. Frequent coexistence of PAIS and FHL tenosynovitis has also been reported.[4,7] This review article describes the diagnostic methods, surgical indications, and surgical techniques for hindfoot endoscopic surgery for PAIS and FHL tendon disorders.

DIAGNOSIS

An important clinical finding of PAIS is a positive hyperplantarflexion test, which is positive when a patient reports posterior ankle pain during forced hyperplantarflexion of the affected ankle. If the test is negative, a diagnosis of PAIS should be ruled out. This clinical test can be substituted for heel-raise standing. Pain behind the medial malleolus is characteristic of FHL tendon disorders and is exacerbated by active or passive ankle and hallux motion. In severe cases of stenosing tenosynovitis, plantar to dorsal flexion of the hallux in the ankle plantar flexion position may reveal crepitus or snapping.

Lateral ankle radiography is useful for detecting abnormalities of the posterolateral talar process, such as an os trigonum or a Stieda process, and CT shows the size and location of such osseous abnormalities in more detail (**Fig. 1**). MRI shows soft tissue abnormalities, including injuries to the posterior capsule and ligament and an inflamed synovium (**Fig. 2**). Effusion of the FHL tendon sheath on MRI is, however, sometimes observed in cases with no symptoms of FHL tendon disorders.[12]

The authors routinely apply ultrasound-guided injection of steroid and local anesthetic to confirm the source of posterior ankle pain. Because PAIS and FHL tendon disorder frequently coexist, ultrasound-guided injection seems necessary not only around the posterolateral talar process but also into the FHL tendon sheath. Ultrasound-guided injections are one type of conservative therapy for PAIS and FHL tendon disorders (**Fig. 3**). Initially, a 1.5-mL injection of 1.0 mL 1% lidocaine mixed with 0.5 mL triamcinolone (40 mg/mL) is given around the posterolateral talar process with ultrasonography and 2 weeks later another injection is given into the FHL tendon sheath.

Although it is important to accurately detect the cause of PAIS or FHL tendon disorders before surgery, it is sometimes difficult in cases accompanied by another

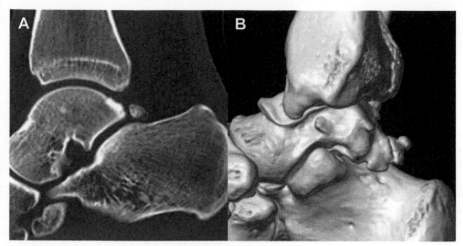

Fig. 1. Sagittal plane CT (*A*) and 3D-CT (*B*) showing an os trigonum.

pathology. To date, the most reliable means for correct diagnosis seems to be hind-foot endoscopy, which enables direct visualization of the pathology.

SURGICAL INDICATIONS

Conservative treatment, including antiinflammatory drugs, ultrasound-guided injection, rest from athletic activity, and physical therapy, is typically the first choice for PAIS and FHL tendon disorders. Hedrick and McBryde[13] reported that nonsurgical treatment was effective in approximately 60% of patients with PAIS. If conservative

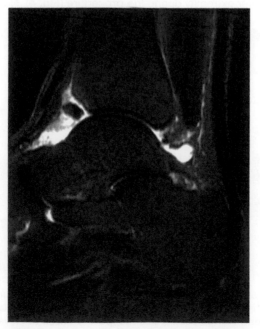

Fig. 2. Sagittal plane MRI showing a soft tissue abnormality of the posterior ankle.

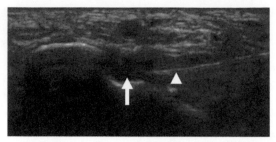

Fig. 3. Ultrasound-guided injection around the posterolateral talar process. (*Arrow*) Os trigonum; (*arrowhead*) injection needle.

treatment fails, however, surgical intervention should be considered. The authors perform conservative treatment exhaustively for 3 months in patients who do not require an early return to athletic activity; for patients who do need to return quickly to sport, the first choice is hindfoot endoscopic surgery.

On the other hand, reported contraindications for hindfoot endoscopic surgery are a localized soft tissue infection (absolute); severe edema; vascular disease, Including diabetic vascular disease; and moderate degenerative joint disease (relative).[14]

SURGICAL TECHNIQUE
Preparation

The patient is placed in the prone position on the operating table under general or spinal anesthesia with the distal 10 cm of the bilateral lower extremities extending beyond the table to enable active dorsal and plantar flexion of the ankle during endoscopic surgery. A small support to elevate the lower leg of the affected extremity up to 10 cm is placed to prevent contact of the arthroscope or instruments with the contralateral lower extremity during the procedure (**Fig. 4**). No distraction device

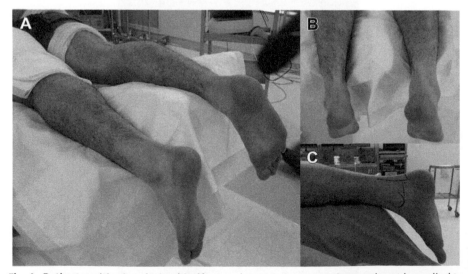

Fig. 4. Patient positioning during hindfoot endoscopy. A pneumatic tourniquet is applied to the upper thigh of the affected extremity (*A*). The distal 10 cm of the bilateral lower extremities are placed beyond the table (*B*). A small support is placed to elevate the lower leg of the affected extremity up to 10 cm (*C*).

is used. A pneumatic tourniquet is applied to the upper thigh of the affected extremity.

Surgical Approach

Hindfoot endoscopy is performed according to van Dijk and colleagues' method.[1] Because slight bleeding in the posterior ankle field prevents the surgeon from performing endoscopic surgery under clear direct visualization, the authors routinely perform hindfoot endoscopy under inflation of the pneumatic tourniquet to elevate systolic blood pressure to at least 120 mm Hg. Two lines are drawn from the tip of the lateral malleolus and medial malleolus to the Achilles tendon, parallel to the sole of the foot. A posterolateral portal and posteromedial longitudinal portal are made between the lines just medial and lateral to the Achilles tendon (**Fig. 5**). Prior to inserting the arthroscope and instruments, a sufficient amount of subcutaneous tissue of the posterior talus is bluntly dissected using mosquito forceps.

Surgical Procedure

A 4.0-mm diameter arthroscope with a 30° angle is inserted through the posterolateral portal toward the second toe and into the extra-articular space of the hindfoot, and a motorized shaver is inserted through the posteromedial portal. The adequate irrigation pressure for saline is approximately 80 mm Hg. First, fatty tissue and scar tissue in the hindfoot are resected using a motorized shaver with a suction apparatus to expose the posterior talus and the FHL tendon. In this procedure, resection is performed by means of soft tissue suction with the cutting edge of the shaver directed posteriorly. If the cutting edge is directed anteriorly before identifying the FHL tendon, there is a risk of iatrogenic injury to the neurovascular bundle. Next, the sliding course of the

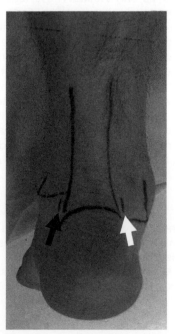

Fig. 5. Posterolateral (*white arrow*) and posteromedial (*black arrow*) portals for hindfoot endoscopy.

FHL tendon is identified to ensure safe endoscopic surgery—this is the most important step in the hindfoot endoscopic technique because the neurovascular bundle lies just medial to this structure. If this process is difficult, passive motion of the great toe under hindfoot endoscopic visualization is helpful for identifying the sliding course of the tendon and exposing it by carefully resecting the overlying soft tissue with forceps or the motorized shaver. As long as the endoscopic procedure is performed in the lateral region of the FHL tendon, there is no risk of iatrogenic injury to the neurovascular bundle. The os trigonum or Stieda process is resected using the motorized shaver while taking care to ensure full removal of any bony prominence compressing the FHL tendon (Video 1). In some cases, a bony prominence can be easily resected using a chisel. In cases of hyperplasia of the synovium on the surface of the FHL tendon, the synovium is resected using forceps. If the FHL tendon is constricted at its entry point into the tarsal tunnel after removing the hypertrophic synovium, the flexor retinaculum is resected to decompress the constricted FHL tendon. After these procedures, smooth sliding of the FHL tendon by passive dorsal and plantar flexion of the ankle and hallux, passive motion of the subtalar joint during passive valgus and varus of the hindfoot, and no residual impingement by passive hyperplantarflexion of the ankle are confirmed under direct visualization on hindfoot endoscopy (Video 2).

COMPLICATIONS

Donnenwerth and Roukis[15] reported in their systematic review of 5 articles (level III and IV studies) that complications occurred in 17 of 452 ankles (3.8%) of 452 patients who underwent hindfoot endoscopy. These included 5 cases with wound-healing problems, 4 with recurrent symptoms, 3 with neuritis of the medial calcaneal nerve, 3 with transient incision anesthesia, and 1 each with traumatic sural neuroma and transient superficial peroneal neuritis; only 8 ankles (1.8%) required additional treatment or operative intervention. Nickisch and colleagues[16] studied the postoperative complications of posterior ankle and hindfoot arthroscopy in 186 ankles of 186 patients. Postoperative complications occurred in 16 ankles (8.5%) and included 4 of plantar numbness, 3 of sural nerve dysesthesia, 4 of Achilles tendon tightness, 2 each of complex regional pain syndrome and infection, and 1 of cyst at the posteromedial portal. Finally, 1 case each of plantar numbness and sural nerve injury failed to resolve. Both these studies revealed a low frequency of complications after hindfoot endoscopy but a high rate of neurologic injuries among the complications that occurred.[15,16] To avoid injury to the sural nerve, the authors recommend making a posterolateral portal just lateral to the Achilles tendon and, to avoid injury to the medial calcaneal nerve, which leads to plantar numbness, advise hindfoot endoscopy in the region lateral to the FHL tendon.

POSTOPERATIVE CARE

An elastic compression bandage is applied to the operated foot without cast immobilization, and the patient is allowed partial weight bearing as tolerated from postoperative day 1. If pain is tolerable, a gradual progression to full weight bearing is permitted. Athletic activity is allowed when the pain has subsided and the full range of motion in the affected foot has returned.

OUTCOMES

Several case series[2–7] have reported the surgical outcomes of posterior ankle disorders treated by hindfoot endoscopy, and most of these studies applied the posterior 2-portal approach introduced by van Dijk and colleagues. Jerosch and Fadel[2] reported the surgical outcomes of 10 athletes who underwent endoscopic resection of a symptomatic os trigonum. As additional procedures, synovectomy of the FHL tendon was performed in 4 cases and release of the tendon sheath was performed in 3.[2] Nine of the 10 patients were symptom-free in activities of daily living within 4 weeks of the surgery and resumed their professional sports activities within 8 weeks. The mean American Orthopedic Foot and Ankle Society (AOFAS) ankle/hindfoot score increased from 43 preoperatively to 87 postoperatively.

Tey and colleagues[3] performed hindfoot endoscopy in 15 ankles of 13 athletes with PAIS who failed to respond to 3 months of conservative treatment and reported that all 15 patients were able to return to full performance with normal plantar flexion at an average of 3 months after surgery. The mean AOFAS hindfoot score improved from 84.4 preoperatively to 98.5 postoperatively, emphasizing the effectiveness of plasty of the posterolateral talus tubercle.

In 2008, Scholten and colleagues[4] investigated the differences in functional outcomes after hindfoot endoscopic surgery for posterior ankle impingement between patients with impingement caused by overuse or trauma and those with osseous or soft tissue impingement. In their 55 patients, the cause of impingement was posttraumatic injury in 36 and overuse in 19. An osseous lesion was removed in 42 patients and a soft tissue lesion was excised in 13. In addition, 63% of the ankle impingement cases were accompanied by FHL tendon disorders. The median time to return to sports activity was 8 weeks (range, 2–15 weeks); however, 13 patients had not returned to sports activities by the final follow-up but with no apparent relationship between the presence of ankle complaints and the cessation of sports activities. The median AOFAS hindfoot score had increased from 75 preoperatively to 90 postoperatively. Although patients in the overuse group were significantly more satisfied at the final follow-up than those in the posttraumatic group, no differences in satisfaction were observed between the osseous and soft tissue impingement groups. The study also revealed a high frequency of coexistence between posterior ankle impingement and FHL tendon disorders.

Willits and colleagues[5] reported the clinical results of posterior ankle arthroscopy for hindfoot impingement in 16 ankles of 15 patients. In their series, all patients were able to return to sporting activities within an average of 5.8 months (range, 1–24 months), and the mean AOFAS score was 91 postoperatively.

In 2013, Smyth and colleagues[7] reported a case series of hindfoot arthroscopic surgery for posterior ankle impingement in which 20 of 22 patients had an os trigonum accompanied by FHL tenosynovitis and the remaining 2 patients had only soft tissue impingement. The mean Foot and Ankle Outcome Score improved significantly from 59 preoperatively to 86 postoperatively, and all patients who reported participating in some level of sporting activity returned to their previous level at a mean of 12 weeks (range, 6–16 weeks) after surgery.[7] Similar to the results of Scholten and colleagues,[4] their study showed the coexistence of posterior ankle impingement and FHL tendon disorders.[7]

SUMMARY

Hindfoot endoscopy through a posterior 2-portal approach is effective both for diagnosis and treatment, enabling direct visualization of posterior ankle pathology with low invasiveness. PAIS, which is generally considered to be a clinical disorder characterized by posterior ankle pain during forced plantar flexion, is the primary indication for hindfoot endoscopic surgery. The most common causes of PAIS are pathologic variants of the posterolateral talar process, such as an os trigonum and a Stieda process, and some studies have reported a high frequency of PAIS coexisting with FHL tendon disorders. Moreover, several studies have reported good clinical outcomes after hindfoot endoscopic surgery for PAIS and FHL tendon disorders. The most important point for achieving good surgical outcomes without major complications is endoscopic identification of the FHL tendon at an early stage in surgery, after which endoscopic procedures should be performed in the region lateral to the FHL tendon to avoid iatrogenic neurovascular injury. Although the reported rate of surgical complications in hindfoot endoscopy is low, most involve nerve injury, particularly to the sural and medial calcaneal nerves. Therefore, surgeons should pay close attention to avoid such complications, especially when making a posterolateral portal or performing surgery before having identified the FHL tendon.

SUPPLEMENTARY DATA

Supplementary data related to this article can be found online at http://dx.doi.org/10.1016/j.fcl.2014.10.005.

REFERENCES

1. van Dijk CN, Scholten PE, Krips RA. 2-portal endoscopic approach for diagnosis and treatment of posterior ankle pathology. Arthroscopy 2000;16(8):871–6.
2. Jerosch J, Fadel M. Endoscopic resection of a symptomatic os trigonum. Knee Surg Sports Traumatol Arthrosc 2006;14(11):1188–93.
3. Tey M, Monllau JC, Centenera JM, et al. Benefits of arthroscopic tuberculoplasty in posterior ankle impingement syndrome. Knee Surg Sports Traumatol Arthrosc 2007;15(10):1235–9.
4. Scholten PE, Sierevelt IN, van Dijk CN. Hindfoot endoscopy for posterior ankle impingement. J Bone Joint Surg Am 2008;90(12):2665–72.
5. Willits K, Sonneveld H, Amendola A, et al. Outcome of posterior ankle arthroscopy for hindfoot impingement. Arthroscopy 2008;24(2):196–202.
6. Ogut T, Ayhan E, Irgit K, et al. Endoscopic treatment of posterior ankle pain. Knee Surg Sports Traumatol Arthrosc 2011;19(8):1355–61.
7. Smyth NA, Murawski CD, Levine DS, et al. Hindfoot arthroscopic surgery for posterior ankle impingement: a systematic surgical approach and case series. Am J Sports Med 2013;41(8):1869–76.
8. Maquirriain J. Posterior ankle impingement syndrome. J Am Acad Orthop Surg 2005;13(6):365–71.
9. Smyth NA, Zwiers R, Wiegerinck JI, et al. Posterior hindfoot arthroscopy: a review. Am J Sports Med 2014;42(1):225–34.
10. Hamilton WG, Geppert MJ, Thompson FM. Pain in the posterior aspect of the ankle in dancers. Differential diagnosis and operative treatment. J Bone Joint Surg Am 1996;78(10):1491–500.
11. Petersen W, Pufe T, Zantop T. Blood supply of the flexor hallucis longus tendon with regard to dancer's tendinitis: injection and immunohistochemical studies of cadaver tendons. Foot Ankle Int 2003;24(8):591–6.
12. Link SC, Erickson SJ, Timins ME. MR imaging of the ankle and foot: normal structures and anatomic variants that may simulate disease. AJR Am J Roentgenol 1993;161(3):607–12.
13. Hedrick MR, McBryde AM. Posterior ankle impingement. Foot Ankle Int 1994;15(1):2–8.

14. van Dijk CN, de Leeuw PA, Scholten PE. Hindfoot endoscopy for posterior ankle impingement. Surgical technique. J Bone Joint Surg Am 2009;91(Suppl 2): 287–98.
15. Donnenwerth MP, Roukis TS. The incidence of complications after posterior hindfoot endoscopy. Arthroscopy 2013;29(12):2049–54.
16. Nickisch F, Barg A, Saltzman CL, et al. Postoperative complications of posterior ankle and hindfoot arthroscopy. J Bone Joint Surg Am 2012;94(5):439–46.

Endoscopic Calcaneoplasty

Joerg Jerosch, MD, PhD*

KEYWORDS

- Calcaneal exostosis • Haglund disease • Endoscopic calcaneoplasty
- Retrocalcaneal bursectomy • Endoscopic surgery

KEY POINTS

- The minimally invasive endoscopic calcaneoplasty is a suitable alternative to the open technique for symptomatic Haglund syndrome.
- Endoscopic calcaneoplasty can achieve reproducible results, allows an excellent differentiation of different disorders, and has fewer complications than the open technique.
- For experienced arthroscopists, the learning curve is short.

INTRODUCTION

Pain in the area of the posterior calcaneus may have different causes, such as paratendonitls, insertional tendinosis of the Achilles, calcaneal apophysitis, retrocalcaneal bursitis, and a Haglund exostosis.[1-21] In 1928, the Swedish orthopedic surgeon, Patrick Haglund,[22] described a syndrome involving a painful osseous prominence of the posterosuperior corner of the calcaneus, large posterior callus, and retrocalcaneal bursitis. The disorder is caused by mechanically induced inflammation of the Achilles tendon and its bursa, from abnormally high pressure between the bursal projection of calcaneus, the Achilles tendon, and the bursal impingement of the Achilles, not by intrinsic tendon disease. Haglund syndrome or disease is often observed bilaterally, mostly at the end of the second or the third decade, and mainly in women. The diagnosis is made with clinical examination and interpretation of radiographs. Hindfoot varus and a pes cavus are both predisposing factors for heel pain because of the vertical position of the calcaneus. Haglund syndrome is also common in athletes. The calcaneal prominence has a hylanized cartilage surface that is contact with the Achilles, and repetitive overuse leads to bursitis and bony hypertrophy.[1]

Disclosures: The author has nothing to disclose.
Department of Orthopedic Surgery and Sports Medicine, Johanna-Etienne-Hospital, Am Hasenberg 46, Neuss 41462, Germany
* Orthopedic Department, Johanna-Etienne-Hospital, Am Hasenberg 46, Neuss 41462, Germany.
E-mail address: j.jerosch@ak-neuss.de

Conservative treatment includes the avoidance of rigid heel counters, activity modification, the use of heel cushions, pads for elevation of the heel, as well as stretching and strengthening of the gastrocnemius-soleus complex. Use of nonsteroidal antiinflammatories and injection of corticosteroids in the retrocalcaneal bursa are also recommended, but direct intratendinous steroid injections may weaken the tendon for at least 14 days, leading in some circumstances to a rupture of the tendon.[23] However, conservative treatment, even over months, may not be effective in some cases and results in high recurrence rates.[24,25]

After failed conservative treatment of more than 6 months, surgical treatment is appropriate.[5,26–28] The traditional approach involves open resection of the dorsolateral edge of the calcaneus, or Haglund prominence, down to the insertion of the Achilles without compromising the tendon. The results after open resection are not always satisfying, and an alternative to the open procedure that can achieve the same goals is the endoscopic calcaneoplasty (ECP).

INDICATIONS/CONTRAINDICATIONS

Patients present with complaints of painful swelling at the level of the Achilles tendon insertion, stiffness, and posterior heel pain with active and passive ankle motion.[5] The posterior heel prominence is often larger and more symptomatic along the posterolateral edge than posteromedially. Retrocalcaneal swelling and pain are often associated, but significant pain and swelling of the distal Achilles insertion site represents tendon disorder and is addressed differently.

Radiographic features seen on a lateral ankle radiograph include a posterior calcaneal exostosis (**Fig. 1**) without intratendinous ossification of the insertion site of the Achilles tendon. Many methods have been proposed in the literature to measure the calcaneal prominence, such as parallel pitch lines or Fowler angle. These methods have been found to have little predictive value and are not useful in clinical practice.[29] The hindfoot is evaluated for alignment and, in patients with hindfoot varus, ECP is not indicated. An apophysitis of the tuber calcanei should also be excluded in juvenile patients.

MRI can show the Haglund exostosis, the extent of the bursa between the Achilles tendon and calcaneus, partial ruptures of the Achilles tendon at the insertion site at the

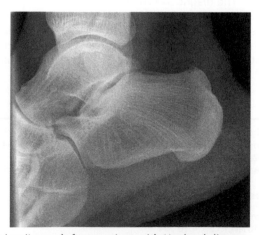

Fig. 1. Typical lateral radiograph for a patient with Haglund disease.

calcaneus, as well as increased intratendinous signal of the Achilles tendon indicating a noninsertional tendinitis (**Figs. 2–4**).

To verify the diagnosis, an injection of a local anesthetic into a painful retrocalcaneal bursa can be useful. ECP is indicated if this test temporarily relieves the symptoms.

Patients should undergo a trial of conservative treatment first. If they do not respond to conservative treatment after 6 months, surgery is indicated.[27,28] However, there are exceptions to this rule. Competitive athletes who cannot perform their athletic activities because of their symptoms may need a surgical solution much earlier.

SURGICAL TECHNIQUE/PROCEDURE
Preoperative Planning

A lateral radiograph in the operation theater is recommended. The patient's skin should be inspected for infection or focal skin lesions, and the vascular status of the operative limb should be checked.

Patient Positioning and Preparation

ECP is generally performed in the supine position under epidural or general anesthesia. An additional local anesthetic block before starting the surgical procedure is helpful to control the postoperative pain. A tourniquet is applied at the thigh and not to the calf. It is placed at the thigh to minimize the risk of neurologic damage to the peroneal nerve, and also to give the surgeon more space when manipulating the instruments.

The affected foot is positioned over the distal edge of the operating table, so that the area of interest can be reached from both sides and be moved freely. The contralateral leg is slightly flexed and abducted on the table so that no interference with the operating field occurs.

For surgical beginners, the prone position may be easier for handling the foot during the operation; it is also safer, with better orientation of the inside structures. Intraoperative radiographic evaluation is also helpful for surgical beginners, until the surgeon feels comfortable with the procedure. Verifying with a c-arm decreases the risk of improper bone resection.

With more experience, the insertion area of the Achilles tendon is an excellent intraoperative landmark, and can easily be identified endoscopically.

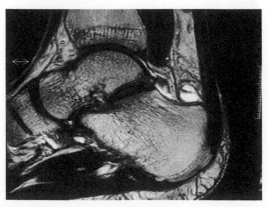

Fig. 2. MRI showing significant retrocalcaneal bursa.

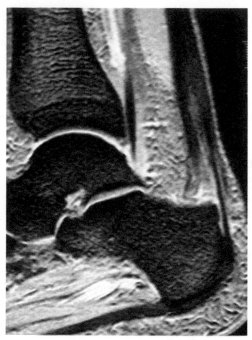

Fig. 3. MRI revealing retrocalcaneal bursa with intratendinous pathologic signal within the Achilles tendon.

Flexion and extension of the ankle is controlled by the surgeon's body, so that adjustment of ankle dorsiflexion can be achieved. With this technique, both hands are free for the instruments and the arthroscope.

The leg is prepped above the knee level and a sterile drape is used about 10 to 15 cm above the ankle (**Fig. 5**).

Surgical Approach

The initial approach can be lateral or medial. I am right handed, and I start with my dominant hand. For establishing the initial portal, a needle is placed directly

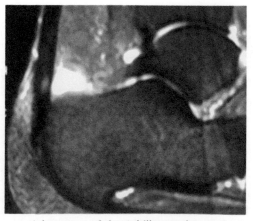

Fig. 4. MRI showing a partial rupture of the Achilles tendon at the insertion site.

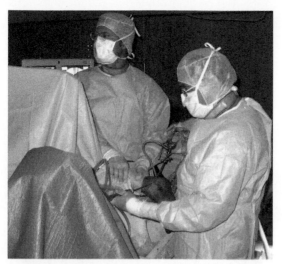

Fig. 5. Patient placement for ECP with c-arm.

at the upper rim of the posterior and superior tip of the calcaneus (**Fig. 6**). This first portal should be located as close as possible to the superior edge of the calcaneus, and also as far posterior as possible. If this portal is too high, it will be difficult later during the procedure to reach the posteroinferior part of the calcaneus.

Fluoroscopic guidance is helpful in order to establish the initial portal. The insertion site of the Achilles tendon is not jeopardized by this approach, because the insertion of the Achilles tendon is much more distal (**Fig. 7**).

A small vertical incision in the skin is made and the subcutaneous tissue is spread by a blunt dissector. We use a standard 4-mm arthroscope, which is positioned in the retrocalcaneal space, as well as a standard-sized instrument for the ECP (**Fig. 8**).

With increasing experience, it is possible to perform the operation without fluoroscopy. Under direct endoscopic control, the contralateral working portal is created using the Wissinger technique (inside out).

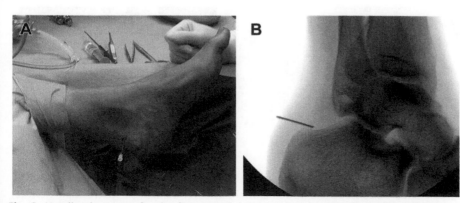

Fig. 6. Needle placement for the first portal. (*A*) Macroscopic view. (*B*) Radiologic view.

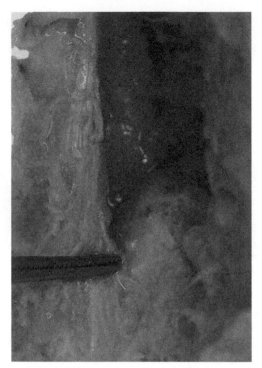

Fig. 7. Distal insertion of the Achilles tendon into the calcaneus.

Surgical Procedure

Step 1

The inflamed retrocalcaneal bursa is identified and resected with a 4-mm resector/shaver (**Fig. 9**). Sometimes there is also significant fibrosis of the bursa, which makes the identification of the bony landmarks difficult.

During resection of the bursa, fibrous tissue, and periosteum short usage of a bipolar resection device can be effective, because less bleeding is expected compared with the immediate use of a traditional shaver. However, prolonged use of a bipolar resection device should be avoided, because the small fluid volume is heated very

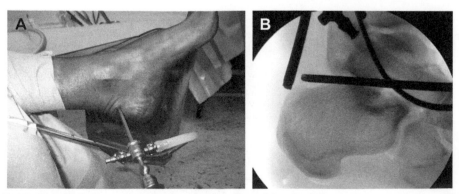

Fig. 8. Standard-size scope and instruments are used for the ECP. (*A*) Macroscopic view. (*B*) Radiologic view.

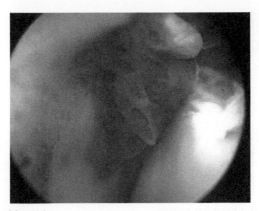

Fig. 9. Retrocalcaneal bursitis.

fast, which can lead to damage to local tissue, including the Achilles tendon, as well as the skin.

Step 2
After the local debridement, the Achilles tendon is localized and prepared. The surface of the calcaneus opposite the Achilles tendon shows a layer of fibrous cartilage (**Fig. 10**). This layer is abraded and the posterior gutter is cleaned completely (**Fig. 11**).

At this step, it necessary to switch the portals so that the bony prominence is completely identified and debrided of the fibrous cartilage, from medial to lateral (**Fig. 12**).

Step 3
The calcaneal exostosis is exposed and resected with the 4-mm burr (**Fig. 13**). The resection starts at one edge (medial or lateral) and is performed as far inferior as possible. It can usually be completed down to the insertion site of the Achilles tendon in the first stages.

At this stage the portals are changed again. Sometimes it may be necessary to change the portal 3 to 4 times before the bony resection is sufficient. It is of special importance to remove the medial and lateral edges of the calcaneus, as well as to smooth down the edges carefully, to prevent leaving bony prominences that might lead to clinical symptoms.

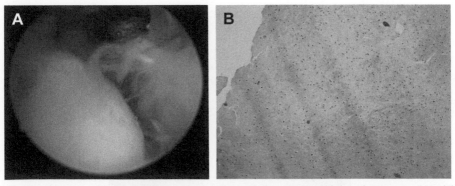

Fig. 10. Fibrous cartilage at the posterior surface of the calcaneus. (*A*) Arthroscopic view. (*B*) HE-staining, magnification ×100.

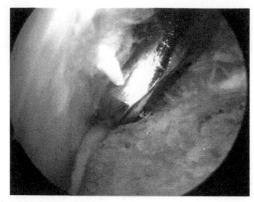

Fig. 11. Cleaning of the posterior gutter.

The arthroscope and the instrument portals are used in an interchangeable manner during the procedure in order to obtain a total bony resection. During the entire procedure the Achilles tendon is protected by the closed side of the burr tip (**Fig. 14**).

Note that the insertion of the Achilles tendon is shaped like a fan and takes hold of the calcaneus in a basketlike configuration (**Fig. 15**). The insertion point of the deep fibers of the Achilles on the posterior aspect of the calcaneus can be visualized and probed during the endoscopic procedure. While resecting the bone, the medial and lateral insertion fibers of the calcaneus are well protected (**Fig. 16**).

Step 4
The insertional area of the Achilles tendon is located distal to the bone spur and, with experience, can safely be exposed (**Fig. 17**). When this area is identified completely from medial to lateral, then bony resection should be sufficient. Arthroscopic images and videos can confirm the extent of the resection and the amount of decompression obtained of the Achilles. As an alternative, lateral radiographs can document the amount of resection.

Step 5
At this stage of the procedure, any disorder of the Achilles tendon should be documented. These disorders can include a yellowish staining of the Achilles tendon, which represents chondroid metaplasia within the tissue (**Fig. 18**).

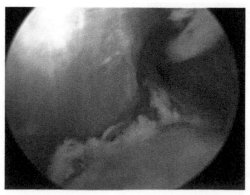

Fig. 12. Preparation of the bony exostosis.

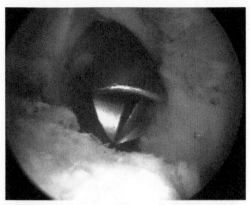

Fig. 13. Bony resection.

Another typical finding is partial tearing of the Achilles tendon from the insertion site. This tearing can range from minimal splitting to an almost subtotal tear (**Fig. 19**). MRI obtained preoperatively should corroborate endoscopic findings (**Fig. 20**). Complete avulsion after ECP has not been reported. However, Achilles tendon avulsions after open resection of a Haglund spur have been described in the literature. The reason for this may be that, with ECP, the surgeon protects the medial and lateral insertional fibers of the Achilles, which protect the tendon, whereas during the open resection the fibers also are released.

Step 6
Any loose tissue, bony debris, and remaining osseous edges are carefully removed with the synovial resector and a thorough flushing with a significant amount of fluid is performed in order to prevent the development of heterotopic ossification.

Step 7
There is no need to place a drain. If a drain is used, this should not be to suction, because this would lead to a significant blood loss (up to 250–350 mL from the cancellous bone of the calcaneus). The skin is carefully closed with 2 to 3 sutures at each incision. A compressive dressing is placed on both sides of the Achilles tendon (**Fig. 21**).

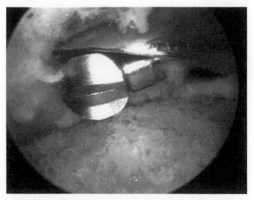

Fig. 14. Protection of the tendon by the closed side of the burr.

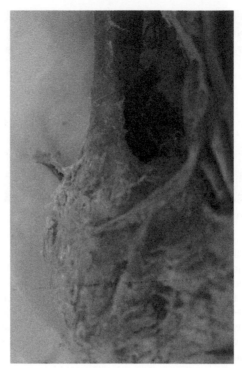

Fig. 15. Anatomic specimen show the medial insertion of the Achilles tendon, which needs to be protected during bone resection.

COMPLICATIONS AND MANAGEMENT

The risk for neurovascular complications is minimal. In one of the first cases, superficial inflammation of the skin was found at the second week, which was thought to be a result of heated irrigation fluid. After 6 weeks, the inflammation resolved. If using a bipolar device in ECP, the surgeon should use a high fluid flow and frequent use of the bipolar device should be minimized. Mechanical instruments should be favored. The

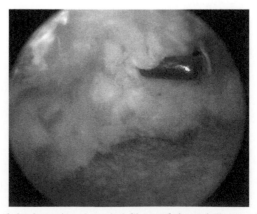

Fig. 16. Protection of the lateral and medial fibers of the Achilles tendon.

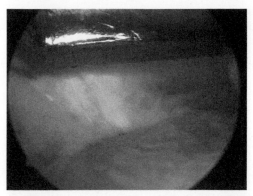

Fig. 17. The distal insertion of the Achilles tendon onto the calcaneus.

small distance between the portals can make endoscopic manipulation difficult, which may increase the risk of injuring the instruments and adjacent structures. Surgeons should be careful to ensure an adequate resection of the calcaneal prominence. Under-resection has been confirmed as the primary reason for persistent postoperative heel pain.[30]

POSTOPERATIVE CARE

Postoperative elevation of the foot for the first 5 to 7 days is recommended. After partial weight bearing for 2 weeks, patients may increase to full weight bearing as tolerated. Normal footwear should not be used for 6 weeks and no athletic activities for at least 12 weeks. After surgery only a minimal swelling is present (**Fig. 22**).

Because of the small portals, the quick subjective satisfaction, and minimal postoperative pain, some patients began early weight bearing against our advice. Some of these patients developed painful local swelling that lasted for several weeks. In 2 cases, the total recovery time was 12 weeks. Therefore, we strictly recommend the use of crutches and partial weight bearing for 2 weeks.

OUTCOMES

With some experience, the intended bony resection can be achieved by the ECP (**Fig. 23**).

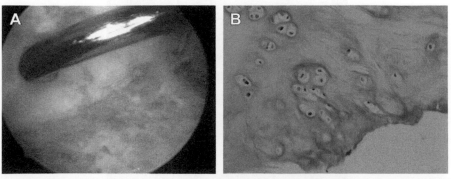

Fig. 18. Yellowish staining of the insertional area of the tendon, representing chondroid metaplasia. (*A*) Arthroscopic view. (*B*) Histological HE-staining, magnification ×100.

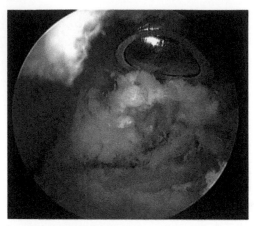

Fig. 19. Endoscopic view. Subtotal avulsion of the Achilles tendon from the calcaneus.

Experienced surgeons can perform the procedure within an operating time of between 15 and 45 minutes (mean, 25 minutes).[31]

Our own experience between 1999 and 2010 in 164 patients (ages, 16–64 years) with an average follow-up of 46.3 months (8–120 months) showed 71 patients with good results and 84 patients with excellent results according to the Ogilvie-Harris score. Only 5 patients showed fair results and 4 patients reported poor results. In 61 patients, preoperative MRI showed a partial rupture of the Achilles tendon close to the insertion site. There were no cases of a complete tear at the time of follow-up. Only minor postoperative complications were observed.

In the open procedure, the surgical goal is to achieve complete exposure of the anatomic site and to perform the resection without weakening the insertion of the Achilles tendon.[7,28,32,33] The same goal can be achieved endoscopically. In the literature, different approaches are mentioned for the open technique, and most of them

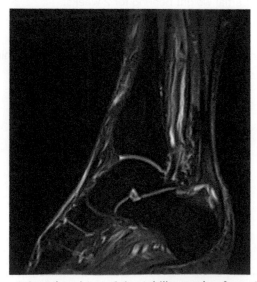

Fig. 20. MRI–imaging. Subtotal avulsion of the Achilles tendon from the calcaneus.

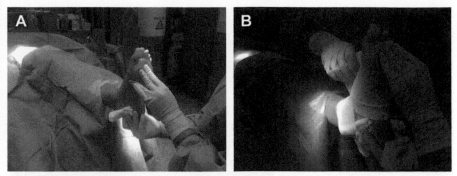

Fig. 21. Postoperative compression bandage. (*A*) Arthroscopic view. (*B*) Close up view.

concur that resection is possible with an incision 1.0 cm medial and longitudinal along the Achilles tendon, which can be prolonged in a J shape.[11] Other investigators prefer bilateral longitudinal incisions adjacent to the Achilles tendon, to completely resect the bony prominence. Another alternative is a direct midline incision followed by a complete central split of the tendons over the whole skin incision length. Debridement of inflammatory or necrotic tissue, as well as the removal of bony tissue, is performed.[11,34]

The results after open Haglund resection and bursectomy vary. In patients with posterior heel pain, resection of the posterosuperior part of the calcaneus and removal of the degenerative and calcified soft tissue leads to good clinical results in about 50% of patients.[2,7,34] Other investigators found an improvement of symptoms in only 69% of patients after bony resection and bursectomy.[33] Our experience with ECP shows good and excellent results in more than 90% of patients.

Following open surgery, various complications have been reported, such as skin complications,[26] Achilles tendon lesions,[35] weakness of the calcaneus after removing the posterosuperior bony prominence,[32] persistent pain,[30] celloid transformation and irritation of the scar (**Fig. 24**),[36] hypesthesia in the area of the scar,[28] and irritation of the whole heel.[30]

The Achilles tendon inserts at the posterior aspect of the calcaneus,[37] where a retrocalcaneal bursa separates the tendon from the calcaneus.[7,8] This anatomy correlates well with the intraoperative endoscopic perspective. Histologic examination of

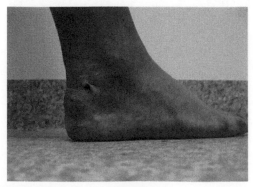

Fig. 22. Swelling observed the day after surgery.

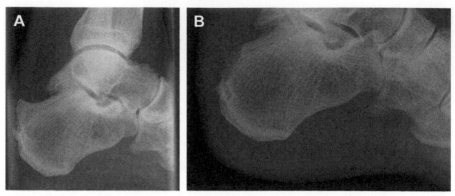

Fig. 23. Preoperative (*A*) and postoperative (*B*) lateral radiographs after ECP.

the anterior bursa, which fits tightly to the calcaneus, shows fibrous cartilaginous tissue; this can also be well documented during calcaneoplasty.

In the posterior part, which is related to the Achilles tendon, an epitenon is described, which cannot be distinguished from the tendon. Biomechanical studies show an increasing pressure on the retrocalcaneal bursa during dorsiflexion of the foot and a decrease of the pressure in plantarflexion. Thus, the main function of the bursa is as a spacer between the axes of the ankle joint and the Achilles tendon.[10,38] The anatomic shape of the superior tuberosity of the calcaneus is variable and ranges from hyperconvex to hypoconvex.[9]

In our experience, clinicians should avoid ECP in patients with bone formation within the distal Achilles tendon insertion. Intrinsic disease of the Achilles tendon cannot be treated endoscopically. For these patients, we suggest a posterior longitudinal incision and a split of the Achilles tendon. After bone resection, the tendon is reattached with either transosseous sutures or bone anchors (**Fig. 25**).

Possible advantages of ECP include reduced morbidity and postoperative pain, earlier rehabilitation, and the possibility of earlier ambulant care.[15–17,29,39]

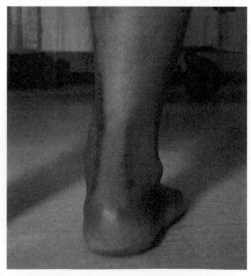

Fig. 24. Scar formation after open surgery.

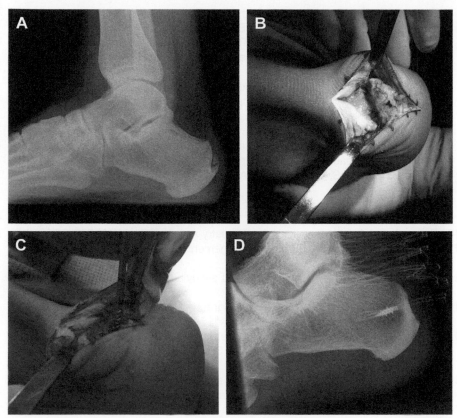

Fig. 25. Resection of an intratendinous ossification with bone anchor fixation. (*A*) Pre operative lateral x-ray. (*B*) Intraoperative situs. (*C*) Placement of the bone anker. (*D*) Postoperative lateral x-ray.

Minimally invasive procedures, including ECP, afford patients lower rates of wound complications and soft tissue healing problems. Our results with ECP compared with the conventional open techniques show fewer complications, earlier rehabilitation, and the accelerated return of patients to their activities after surgery. Surgeons who are familiar with arthroscopic surgery will soon prefer ECP to open Haglund resection.

SUMMARY

The minimally invasive ECP is a suitable alternative to the open technique for symptomatic Haglund syndrome. ECP can achieve reproducible results, allows an excellent differentiation of different disorders, and benefits from fewer complications than the open technique. For experienced arthroscopists, the learning curve is short.

REFERENCES

1. Clancy WO. Runners' injuries. Part two. Evaluation and treatment of specific injuries. Am J Sports Med 1980;8:287–9.
2. Fiamengo SA, Warren RF, Marshall JL, et al. Posterior heel pain associated with a calcaneal step and Achilles tendon calcification. Clin Orthop 1982;167:203–11.

3. Fowler A, Philip JF. Abnormality of the calcaneus as a cause of painful heel: its diagnosis and operative treatment. Br J Surg 1945;32:494–8.
4. Frey C, Rosenberg Z, Shereff MJ. The retrocalcaneal bursa: anatomy and bursography. Am Orthop Foot and Ankle Society Specialty Day Meeting. Las Vegas, February 15, 1989.
5. Heneghan JA, Pavlov H. The Haglund painful heel syndrome. Experimental investigation of cause and therapeutic implications. Clin Orthop 1984;187:228–34.
6. Jones DC, James SL. Partial calcaneal osteotomy for retrocalcaneal bursitis. Am J Sports Med 1984;12:72–3.
7. Keck SW, Kelly PJ. Bursitis of the posterior part of the heel: evaluation of surgical treatment of 18 patients. J Bone Joint Surg Am 1965;47A:267–73.
8. Leach RE, James S, Wasilewski S. Achilles tendinitis. Am J Sports Med 1981;9:93–8.
9. Mann RA, editor. DuVries surgery of the foot. 5th edition. St Louis (MO): Mosby; 1986.
10. Ruch JA. Haglund's disease. J Am Podiatry Assoc 1974;64:1000–3.
11. Schepsis AA, Leach RE. Surgical management of Achilles tendinitis. Am J Sports Med 1987;15:308–15.
12. Hartmann HO. The tendon sheaths and synovial bursae of the foot. Foot Ankle 1981;1:247–96.
13. Burhenne LJ II, Connell DG. Xeroradiography in the diagnosis of the Haglund syndrome. J Can Assoc Radiol 1986;37:157–60.
14. Jerosch J, Steinbeck J, Schröder M, et al. Arthroscopic treatment of anterior synovitis of the ankle in athletes. Knee Surg Sports Traumatol Arthrosc 1994;2:176–81.
15. Jerosch J, Steinbeck J, Schröder M, et al. Arthroscopically assisted arthrodesis (AAA) of the ankle joint. Arch Orthop Trauma Surg 1996;115:182–9.
16. Jerosch J. Arthroskopische Operationen am oberen Sprunggelenk. Indikationen, Technik, Ergebnisse, Komplikationen. Orthopade 1999;28:538–49.
17. Jerosch J. Endoscopic release of plantar fasciitis - a benign procedure. Foot Ankle Int 2000;21:511–3.
18. Pavlov H, Heneghan MA, Hersh A. The Haglund syndrome: initial and differential diagnosis. Radiology 1982;144:83–8.
19. Ogilvie-Harris DJ, Mahomed N, Demaziere A. Anterior impingement of the ankle treated by arthroscopic removal of bony spurs. J Bone Joint Surg Br 1993;75B:437–40.
20. Stephens MM. Haglund's deformity and retrocalcaneal bursitis. Orthop Clin North Am 1994;25:41–6.
21. Leitze Z, Sella EJ, Aversa JM. Endoscopic decompression of the retrocalcaneal space. J Bone Joint Surg Am 2003;85-A:1488–96.
22. Haglund P. Beitrag zur Klinik der Achilles tendon. Zeitschr Orthop Chir 1928;49:49–58.
23. Kennedy JC, Willis RB. The effects of local steroid injections on tendons: a biomechanical and microscopic correlative study. Am J Sports Med 1976;4:11–21.
24. Jerosch J, Nasef NM. Endoscopic calcaneoplasty – rationale, surgical technique, and early results: a preliminary report. Knee Surg Sports Traumatol Arthrosc 2003;11:190–5.
25. van Dijk CN, van Dyk CE, Scholten PE, et al. Endoscopic calcaneoplasty. Foot Ankle Clin 2006;2:439–46.
26. Angermann P. Chronic retrocalcaneal bursitis treated by resection of the calcaneus. Foot Ankle 1990;10:285–7.

27. Ippolito E, Ricciardi-Pollini PT. Invasive retrocalcaneal bursitis: a report on three cases. Foot Ankle 1984;4:204–8.
28. Pauker M, Katz K, Yosipovitch Z. Calcaneal osteotomy for Haglund's disease. J Foot Surg 1992;31:558–89.
29. Jardé O, Quenot P, Trinquier-Lautard JL, et al. Haglund disease treated by simple resection of calcaneus tuberosity. An angular and therapeutic study. Apropos of 74 cases with 2 years follow-up. Rev Chir Orthop Reparatrice Appar Mot 1997; 83(6):566–73.
30. Nesse E, Finsen V. Poor results after resection for Haglund's heel. Analysis of 35 heels treated by arthroscopic removal of bony spurs. Acta Orthop Scand 1994; 65(1):107–9.
31. Jerosch J, Sokkar S, Dücker M, et al. Endoscopic calcaneoplasty (ECP) in Haglund's syndrome. Indication, surgical technique, surgical findings and results. Z Orthop Unfall 2012;150:250–6.
32. Periman MD. Enlargement of the entire posterior aspect of the calcaneus: treatment with the Keck and Kelly calcaneal osteotomy. J Foot Surg 1992;31:424–33.
33. Schnieder W, Niehus W, Knahr K. Haglund's syndrome: disappointing results following surgery: a clinical and radiographic analysis. Foot Ankle Int 2000; 21(1):26–30.
34. McGarvey WC, Sparks M, Baxter DE. Causes of heel pain. The rational approach to diagnosis, management, and salvage of complications. Foot Ankle Clin 1998; 3:175–87.
35. Le TA, Joseph PM. Common exostectomies of the rearfoot. Clin Podiatr Med Surg 1991;8:601–23.
36. Leach RE, Dilorio E, Harney RA. Pathological hindfoot conditions in the athlete. Clin Orthop 1983;177:116–21.
37. Goss CM. Gray's anatomy. 27th edition. Philadelphia: Lea & Febiger; 1959. p. 544–53.
38. Canoso JJ, Liu N, Trall MR, et al. Physiology of the retrocalcaneal bursa. Ann Rheum Dis 1988;47:910–2.
39. Jerosch J, Schunck J, Sokkar SH. Endoscopic calcaneoplasty (ECP) as a surgical treatment of Haglund's syndrome. Knee Surg Sports Traumatol Arthrosc 2007; 15:927–34.

Index

Note: Page numbers of article titles are in **boldface** type.

Foot Ankle Clin N Am 20 (2015) 167–193
http://dx.doi.org/10.1016/S1083-7515(15)00009-1
1083-7515/15/$ – see front matter © 2015 Elsevier Inc. All rights reserved.

foot.theclinics.com

Moving?

Make sure your subscription moves with you!

To notify us of your new address, find your **Clinics Account Number** (located on your mailing label above your name), and contact customer service at:

Email: journalscustomerservice-usa@elsevier.com

800-654-2452 (subscribers in the U.S. & Canada)
314-447-8871 (subscribers outside of the U.S. & Canada)

Fax number: 314-447-8029

Elsevier Health Sciences Division
Subscription Customer Service
3251 Riverport Lane
Maryland Heights, MO 63043

*To ensure uninterrupted delivery of your subscription, please notify us at least 4 weeks in advance of move.

Printed and bound by CPI Group (UK) Ltd, Croydon, CR0 4YY

07/10/2024

01040499-0019